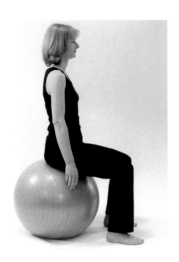

Collins need to know?

Pilates

D1426308

DORSET COUNTY LIBRARY

204264235 S

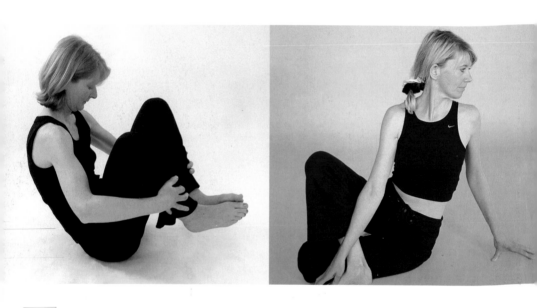

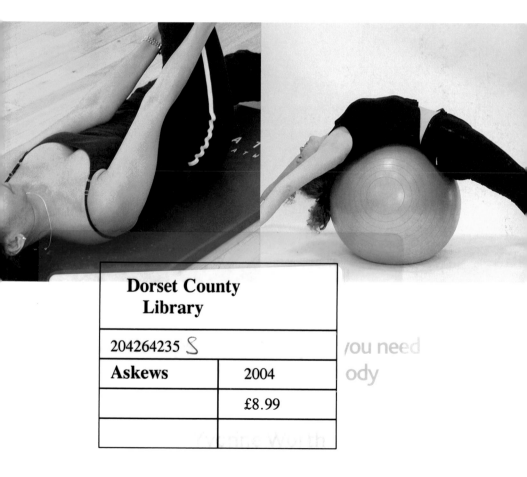

Collins need to know?

Pilates

Dorset County Library		
204264235 S		
Askews	2004	
	£8.99	

/ou need

ody

First published in 2004 by
Collins, an imprint of
HarperCollins*Publishers*
77–85 Fulham Palace Road
Hammersmith, London W6 8JB

The Collins website address is: www.collins.co.uk

Collins is a registered trademark of HarperCollins*Publishers* Limited

09 08 07 06 05 04
6   5   4   3   2   1

Text and illustrations © The Printer's Devil, 2003; HarperCollins*Publishers*, 2004
Design © HarperCollins*Publishers*, 2004

The majority of photographs in this book were taken by Focus Publishing.

All rights reserved. No part of this publication may be reproduced, stored in a retrieval system, or transmitted, in any form or by any means, electronic, mechanical, photocopying, recording or otherwise, without the prior written permission of the publishers.

A catalogue record for this book is available from the British Library

Created by: Focus Publishing, Sevenoaks, Kent
Project editor: Guy Croton
Editor: Vanessa Townsend
Designer: David Etherington
Project co-ordinator: Caroline Watson
Front cover photograph: © Getty Images/David Sacks
Cover design: Cook Design

ISBN 0 00 719063 8

Colour reproduction by Colourscan, Singapore
Printed and bound by Printing Express Ltd, Hong Kong

The information contained in this book, including addresses, telephone numbers and website details, is correct at the time of going to press but the publisher cannot accept responsibility for any subsequent changes.

It is advisable to consult your doctor before starting any exercise regime. The author and publisher do not accept liability for any injury suffered as a result of negligence in performing the exercises contained in this book. Exercises contained in this book are carried out at your own risk and may not be suitable for every reader.

contents

pilates

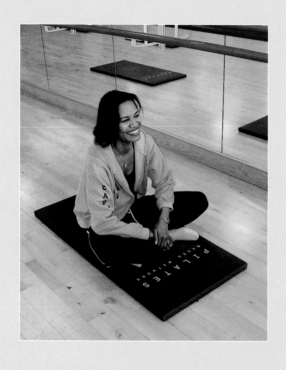

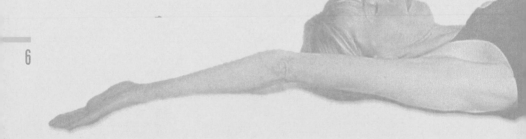

basics

If you are looking for a form of exercise and an enjoyable pastime that will make you feel good, then Pilates could be for you. This well established and acclaimed form of body conditioning is now practised regularly by millions of people all around the world. It requires next to no equipment, only average levels of fitness and a positive approach.

▶ What is Pilates?

The Pilates technique is a unique system of body conditioning that stretches and strengthens the muscles, as well as improving flexibility, balance, breathing, posture and alignment.

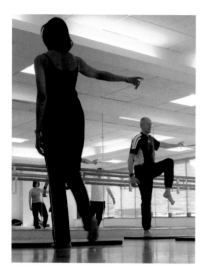

▲ Most leisure and sports centres offer Pilates courses for different levels of ability from beginner to advanced.

Pilates trains you to recognize your strengths and your weaknesses, while providing you with the means of correcting those weaknesses, thereby strengthening and rebalancing your entire body mechanism. Many other exercise systems work primarily on strengthening the muscles themselves, focussing largely on working the limbs. Pilates, on the other hand, concentrates on strengthening the central core and using the abdominal muscles to control the different movements: it also encourages you to focus your mind as you exercise the body, gradually improving your general awareness, co-ordination and overall alignment.

The Pilates system of exercise, which dates back to the mid-1920s, was an unusual approach to exercise in the West at the time. Drawing its influences from Western and Eastern influences alike, it advocated not only the need for regular physical exercise, but also the necessity of bringing our lives into balance on all levels – insisting that we eat a healthy diet, get plenty of sleep, reduce stress in our lives and hold a positive attitude in all matters.

Pilates today

Today, the growing interest in maintaining an holistic lifestyle, sustaining a level of health and fitness and achieving a sense of wellbeing in body, mind and spirit, has led to an increasing popularity in the principles and practice of Pilates.

A further reason for the current popularity of the Pilates system is its potential to change the

WATCH OUT!

Basic fitness

All forms of exercise require a basic level of fitness. Although Pilates movements need not be especially strenuous, if in any doubt you should check with your doctor before embarking on a course.

body shape. Pilates works to stretch and lengthen the muscles, encouraging the body to become stronger and firmer, but without the disadvantage of also building unwanted bulk. The technique also works to improve posture, thereby allowing you to use your body more effectively and efficiently, even when carrying out mundane daily activities.

Moreover, Pilates does not require you to give up your current fitness routine. Quite the opposite, it was always intended as a system that would work in conjunction with other exercise programmes: strengthening, rebalancing and realigning the body, while also improving body awareness and therefore reducing the risk of strain or injury that can so easily occur in many other forms of exercise. Indeed, Pilates is recommended as a complement to other exercises, not a substitute: even the most dedicated Pilates student is advised to also incorporate some form of cardiovascular exercise into his or her weekly routine.

MUST KNOW

Fitness for all
Because the exercises are all adaptable to the needs of the individual, a major attraction of Pilates is that it is suitable for anyone, regardless of age, size or level of fitness. It is also beneficial to those who wish to rehabilitate physically.

▼ Pilates is an excellent complementary discipline that will improve your flexibility for other sports.

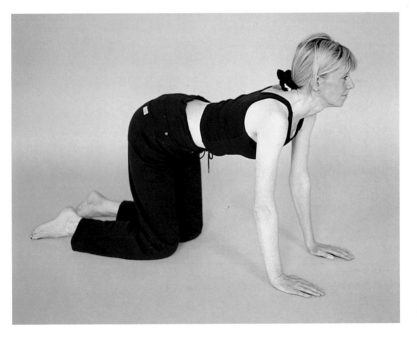

PILATES BASICS

9

History of Pilates

Founded in the early twentieth century by a German fitness fanatic, the Pilates technique was an extraordinarily progressive and unusually holistic approach to exercise for its time.

Joseph Hubertus Pilates was born in 1880, near Dusseldorf in Germany. As a child he was extremely frail, suffering from various conditions, including rickets, asthma and even rheumatic fever. Determined to overcome his ill health and lead a healthy life, he engaged in a programme of rigorous exercise, exploring various disciplines and activities, including gymnastics, body-building, wrestling, diving and skiing. Taking selected elements from various different activities he devised a programme of fitness that would help him achieve his maximum possible level of fitness, strength and flexibility.

In 1912 Pilates, aged 32, decided to move to the UK, where he earned his living as a boxer, circus performer and a self-defence instructor to detectives. During the First World War he was taken prisoner, due to his German identity. Interned in a camp on the Isle of Man, his duties in the hospital gave him the opportunity to reconsider his fitness routine, adapting the exercises to the various needs of his fellow inmates.

After the war Joseph Pilates returned to Germany, where he continued to develop his fitness system. Initially he was employed to work with the local police force but eventually he was drafted into the army. In 1926, unable to tolerate the political climate in Germany any longer, he set sail for America. On board ship he met a young woman, Clara, who would later become his wife.

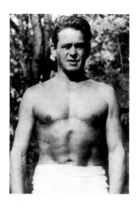

▲ Joseph Pilates' unique method first gained popularity in America during the 1920s.

MUST KNOW

Origins of Pilates
Joseph Pilates' original set of exercises, developed in the 1920s, was made up of 34 basic moves and manifests influences from Eastern and Western disciplines alike – the natural result of Joseph's years of pursuing many different methods of exercise and fitness.

Once in New York, Joseph, with Clara's help, set about establishing his first exercise studio. The location was 939 Eighth Avenue. Very little is known about the studio's early years, but by the 1940s Pilates had achieved great popularity in the performance world with his extraordinary technique – dancers, gymnasts, athletes and actors alike were drawn to his studio, including young ballerinas at the NYC Ballet.

In the past few decades the Pilates technique has continued to grow in popularity, both with professionals for whom fitness is a vital part of their working life and with those members of the general public who have an interest in fitness and well-being.

Pilates himself advocated that, along with an ongoing commitment to regular exercise, each of us should be prepared to examine and alter the various aspects of our daily lives and work towards improving our overall fitness and sense of well-being, both physically and mentally.

MUST KNOW

Philosophy of Pilates

Pilates' routine did not simply consist of a particular set of physical movements to be repeated mindlessly: a fundamental element in the philosophy of Pilates is that true fitness and well-being can only be achieved through a complete integration of the mind and the body.

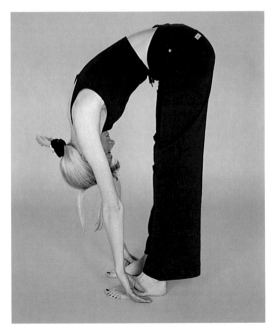

◄ The popularity of Pilates has boomed in recent years. The basic principles of the technique remain unchanged, but methods of teaching vary in style and emphasis according to the individual needs of its exponents.

Physiology

Fundamental to the teachings of Pilates is an understanding and appreciation of human physiology. One of the chief aims of the discipline is to maximize the body's natural potential.

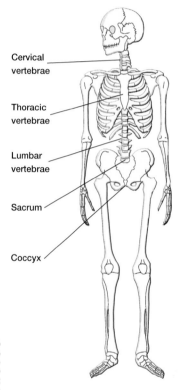

Cervical vertebrae

Thoracic vertebrae

Lumbar vertebrae

Sacrum

Coccyx

Skeleton, bones & joints

The spine (or vertebral column), skull, ribs and sternum make up the axial skeleton. The spinal column is comprised of 33 bones, known as vertebrae: seven cervical vertebrae (the neck); 12 thoracic vertebrae (the upper back); five lumbar vertebrae (the lower back); five sacral vertebrae, which are fused together to make one bone called the sacrum (located at the base of the spine), and four coccygeal vertebrae, which are fused into one or two bones called the coccyx (the tailbone). The vertebrae are separated from each other by intervertebral discs, which are made up of fibrocartilaginous material.

The natural shape of the spinal column is actually a slight 'S'. The spine itself both supports the weight of the body and gives the body its basic posture. It also provides protection for the spinal cord and spinal nerve roots. The natural curves of the spine and the intervertebral discs allow the spine to function

> **WATCH OUT!**
>
> ### Look after your back
>
> The spinal column – especially the neck – is a highly sensitive part of the body that should never be put under undue stress during exercise. If you have suffered from back or neck problems in the past, or have sustained any injuries to the spine, check with your doctor or physiotherapist before embarking on a course of Pilates.

rather like a spring, making action more agile and absorbing any shock impact to the body. When the spinal curves are altered in any way (for example, repeatedly sitting in an uncomfortable, badly aligned position), stresses are placed on the spine that can lead to bad posture and, eventually, to pain.

The muscles of the body

The central section of any muscle is made up of bundles of thin, parallel fibres, surrounded by a layer of connective tissue. Each muscle fibre has a nerve ending (motor end plate), which receives messages from the brain instructing the muscle to contract. In instances of major muscle movement, such as in the large thigh muscles, one nerve ending will serve numerous muscle fibres, whereas, for fine movements, such as delicate movements of the fingers, a single nerve ending will supply only a few fibres.

Muscle fibres function in a very simple manner – they are either 'switched on'

MUST KNOW

Muscle tone
Good muscle tone will improve your posture and should give you an enhanced sense of well-being. Pilates stretches and lengthens muscles as well as strengthening them, which makes them look as well as feel good. With regular exercise many students start to see and feel the benefits very quickly.

▼ The Pilates technique offers an excellent workout for all the different muscle groups.

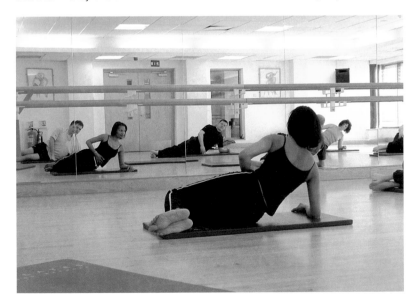

PILATES BASICS

13

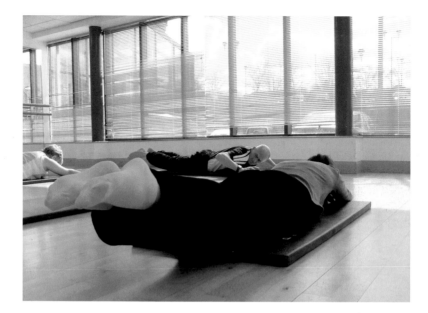

(stimulated) or 'switched off' (not stimulated). Therefore, the degree of muscular contraction is not dependent upon the extent of the fibre stimulation, but upon the actual number of fibres stimulated – the more fibres that are 'switched on', the greater the degree of contraction.

Equally, muscles cannot push, they can only pull, and so the only way they are able to function effectively is by working in opposing pairs. When one pair of muscles contracts, or shortens, the other pair relaxes, or stretches. This system creates the body's ability to move.

▲ If you start to feel any 'twinges' in the middle of any exercise, stop immediately. This is your muscles' way of telling you that you are pushing yourself too far too quickly.

The stretch reflex

The muscle is provided with a protective mechanism called a stretch reflex. This mechanism is triggered when any muscle is stretched too quickly. Each muscle contains cells that are known as 'muscle spindles'. When a muscle is stretched too fast, and is

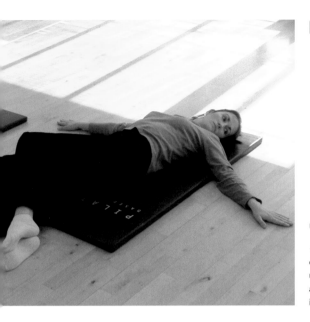

MUST KNOW

Keep your muscles warm
Warm muscles work more efficiently
and effectively than cold ones and
are less likely to 'pull' or 'tear'. For
this reason it is vital to warm up
before any kind of exercise –
particularly that which includes
moves that thoroughly stretch the
muscles. See pages 32–45 for a full
warm-up programme for Pilates.

◀ It is essential to include a
cool down as well as a warm-
up into your exercise routine
and to ease the body gently
into any stretching position.

therefore at risk of tearing, the muscle's
spindles are activated, automatically triggering
the muscle concerned to contract and
thereby avoiding injury to the muscle. It is for
this reason that, when exercising, it is
essential for us to ease into any stretching
movement slowly and gradually.

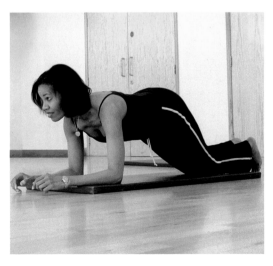

▶ As your muscles become
stronger, you will find that
you have greater control and
can hold positions longer.

Principles of Pilates

Joseph Pilates' exercise system was built around 34 moves, backed by a set of basic principles designed to maximize harmony between the mind and body.

Concentration

The Pilates technique is not a system of mindlessly repeated exercises in which your body runs on automatic while your mind switches off completely. On the contrary, exercising under the Pilates system requires a great deal of focus and concentration. The mind and body must work together, with the mind remaining alert as each aspect of every movement is carefully controlled and monitored.

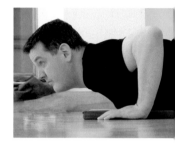

▲ To make the most of Pilates, focus your attention on what you are doing – the movement and your breathing – and try to avoid letting your mind wander.

Control

In order for us to maintain correct posture and alignment as we work the various different muscles, it is essential for us to acquire good muscle control. In Pilates we exercise to strengthen the body by working against gravity using slow and controlled movements – the slower we are able to work any particular movement, while keeping the move controlled, the stronger the body will gradually become.

Breathing

Correct execution of the Pilates exercises requires us to use appropriate breathing. Many people have learned to hold their breath as they exercise, or to take shallow breaths into the upper chest, causing a build-up of tension in the body, inhibiting the supply of oxygen to the muscles and reducing the performance of the muscles. In Pilates we breathe deeply, into the lower ribs and the back, moving our muscles in a slow, even rhythm in time with the breathing.

MUST KNOW

Breathe deeply
Using the breath as you move will also help ensure that your movements are smooth, controlled and rhythmic.

Centring

The body's centre, or centre of gravity, is also referred to as the central or abdominal core, or even, sometimes, the powerhouse. The Pilates system considers the body's place of power and control to be here, at the body's centre of gravity (an area approximately 5cm/2in below the navel, also known in some disciplines as the 'hara'). Under the Pilates system, all moves are controlled by the contraction of the muscles located here – the abdominal muscles: if we work from this central core we learn to lengthen and stretch our muscles without risk of strain or injury.

Precision

The effectiveness of the Pilates exercises relies on precise execution of each move, and this can only be achieved with a great deal of concentration, patience and practice. As with any new discipline, when you start learning Pilates it can be extremely difficult to remember the various different points, but, with practice, controlling your muscles while keeping your abdominals contracted and your spine in neutral, and stretching and lengthening your muscles in rhythm with your breathing, will start to occur automatically.

Flowing movements

The aim with all the Pilates exercises is to make them as even and flowing as possible, without jarring or jerky movements. Each of the sequences or repetitions of the moves should be controlled throughout by the abdominals and performed using a continuous, slow, smooth, flowing movement, in rhythm with the breathing.

Awareness

A keen awareness of the different parts of our physical body is essential if we are to perform the various Pilates moves effectively.

WATCH OUT!

Correct technique
Learning to maintain the abdominal contraction (page 31) – thereby gradually improving the body's core strength – is an essential aspect of the Pilates method.

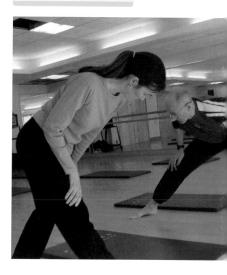

▲ Always listen to your body as you practise the moves. Increased bodily awareness will ensure greater control and efficiency.

Pilates for you

The Pilates system of exercise can be easily adapted to suit your own particular schedule and preferences. The matwork movements provide you with a thorough programme of exercises, which can be done in the privacy of your own home.

Courses and classes

You can, of course, successfully work out at home, but, if you find that you would prefer not to exercise on your own, or you simply decide that you would like to work under the guidance of a qualified instructor or expand your knowledge of the Pilates technique, there are many excellent courses and classes available to you. You have the choice of going to a specialist Pilates studio, of which there are many, or attending some of the various classes on offer at a large number of sports, fitness and leisure centres. The majority of Pilates teachers will also give you the option of either group or private sessions.

WATCH OUT!

Make it count
To have any real effect, Pilates should be practised for a minimum of one hour a week, but how you choose to do this is entirely up to you.

▼ Many sports and leisure centres offer Pilates group classes with a specialist teacher.

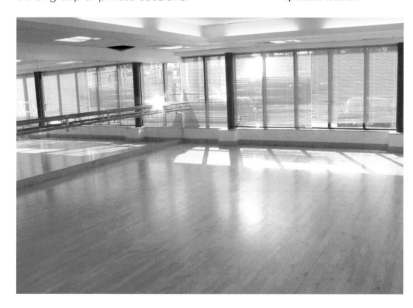

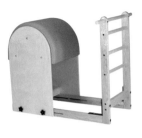
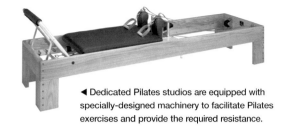

◄ Dedicated Pilates studios are equipped with specially-designed machinery to facilitate Pilates exercises and provide the required resistance.

Learning with an experienced Pilates instructor to guide you is extremely beneficial, as they are fully qualified to assess your particular needs and will be able to guide you and monitor your progress. So, even if your intention is to work out at home, you might consider enrolling on at least a short course of Pilates classes or even taking some one-to-one sessions.

Working with equipment

Joseph Pilates' original routine consisted of a mixture of exercises, some of which would be done on the floor and others that would be performed using his specially designed exercise equipment. Nowadays, many teachers work purely using matwork exercises, with the aid of some very simple pieces of equipment, such as tennis balls and rubber exercise bands, but there is also the option of attending a well-equipped Pilates studio and working with the exercise machinery too. This is rather like visiting a gym, although the equipment is quite different in design and many of the machines use springs, rather than weights, to provide you with added resistance as you exercise. The atmosphere of most Pilates studios is also very different to that of a regular gym, tending to be calm and stress-free, frequently with relaxing music playing in the background. Also, students always work under the strict guidance of a qualified instructor.

Books, videos and dvds

With the rapidly growing popularity of the Pilates technique, there is an ever-increasing number of excellent books, videos and DVDs available today (some of which are listed on pages 186–7). These will give you the opportunity to learn more about Pilates and the different approaches and give you the chance to develop your exercise routine to suit your own needs and preferences. The approach of different instructors can vary, as each may choose to focus on a slightly different system or element of the Pilates method – some even combine Pilates with other disciplines, such as yoga or the Alexander Technique.

Practising Pilates

Every form of exercise has a few golden rules that should be observed, and Pilates is no exception. Very little specialist equipment is required, but it pays to heed the following advice.

Safety

Most fitness systems these days recognize the importance of safety and have taken steps to make sure that risk of strain or injury is avoided wherever possible. However, many of the injuries that we suffer tend not to occur on the sports field or in the gym, but as we go about our daily activities – muscles can be pulled while lifting small children, bags of shopping or even picking up a toothbrush. The Pilates technique totally retrains the body, improving posture, balance and alignment, and increasing strength, flexibility, stability and muscle control. The result of this is that we are better able to carry out our everyday activities without risk of injury.

> **WATCH OUT!**
>
> **Be realistic**
> If you have never exercised regularly before, or have not followed a regime for a long time, be realistic in your expectations of your basic fitness.

Self-awareness

The increased self-awareness that the Pilates system encourages makes us more mindful of exactly how we are using our bodies, enabling us to recognize bad habits, thus giving us the opportunity to change them. A growing self-awareness also allows us to identify any areas that require attention, so letting us strengthen and improve our weak spots.

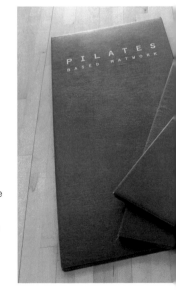

Equipment

The Pilates technique does not necessarily require you to buy any special clothing or equipment, although various types of equipment are available should you choose to purchase them.

To practise Pilates, make sure you are wearing comfortable clothing that allows you to move freely. Remember, Pilates is not a particularly strenuous type of exercise and therefore, certainly to begin with, you will need to make sure that you are wearing sufficient clothing to keep you warm as you exercise.

The only pieces of equipment that you require are:

- a folded towel, blanket or exercise mat to place on the floor to protect you as you exercise;
- a scarf or stretchy rubber exercise band;
- a flat cushion, or small folded towel to place under your head, if necessary.

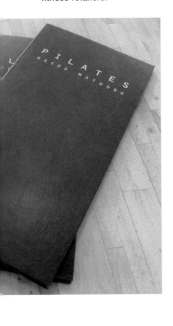

▼ Special mats that are designed for Pilates exercises are available from many sports and fitness retailers.

MUST KNOW

The benefits of Pilates

- Improves mind/body awareness.
- Develops the body's core abdominal strength.
- Increases strength and improves balance.
- Lengthens and stretches the muscles to give you a leaner body without building bulk.
- Reduces stress levels and fatigue.
- Improves stability, flexibility and joint mobility.
- Reduces incidences of strain and injury.
- Boosts the immune system.
- Gives an increased sense of well-being.
- Improves circulation and muscle tone.
- Enhances muscle control without causing tension.
- Improves the functioning of the respiratory and lymphatic systems.
- Relieves headaches and can help eliminate the cause of stress-, tension-, or posture-related headaches.
- Improves bone density.
- Relieves pain, stiffness and tension.
- Exercises the muscles without causing pain or risking muscle tears or strains or jarred joints
- Teaches you to enjoy the movements as you stretch.
- Is suitable for anyone, regardless of age or level of fitness.
- The fundamental principles of the Pilates method can be applied to any movement or activity.

Pilates for a healthy body

Plan your exercise routine to suit your lifestyle and be realistic about what you will actually be able to achieve. Is it easier and more efficient for you to exercise for a few minutes each day, rather than one long weekly session? Or would a longer session suit you better?

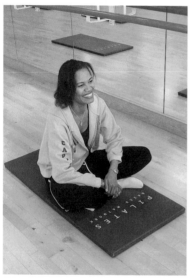

▲ Pilates will give you a greater sense of well-being – so long as you don't overdo it...

Organize a programme of exercise for yourself that you will easily be able to fulfil each week: there is no point in setting yourself impossible goals that only leave you feeling frustrated when you are unable to meet them, or that push you too hard and leave you feeling exhausted and burnt out.

The most important factor is your willingness to commit to a regular exercise programme (regardless of how much or little time you have available), and to make positive changes in your daily life. Only with consistent practice will you truly begin to notice lasting changes to your body shape, your fitness levels, your health and your feeling of well-being. Remember, though, the more you exercise the quicker you will see the results and the more benefit you will feel.

For Pilates to effect real and lasting changes you need to dedicate a total time of at least an hour each week to the exercise.

Best time to exercise

Choose a time to exercise when you will not be continually interrupted, and unplug the telephone. You might even like to put on some relaxing background music. If you are someone who finds it hard to prioritize taking time to do things for yourself, and constantly find yourself intending to exercise, but always being pulled away to do something else, you might even consider booking an 'appointment' with yourself in advance for a specific time and day, which you do not allow yourself to cancel or change.

Noticing the effects

Some people notice immediate changes with Pilates, but it usually takes around six to ten sessions for most people to start to notice an overall improvement in their posture, body shape, stamina, strength and flexibility.

Planning your exercise routine

In principle, the ideal time to exercise is at the end of the day, when your muscles are warmed up. But the best time to choose is the one that appeals to you most and fits best with your schedule – maybe the start of the day is the optimum time for you to exercise, preparing you for the day ahead; or perhaps you favour a relaxing wind-down in the evening, to help you let go of the stresses and strains of a hectic day.

If you choose to exercise first thing in the morning, start by rolling down against a wall (page 35) a few times, to help mobilize your spine and gently wake up the whole body.

If you exercise in the evening, it is a good idea to begin your sessions by lying on your back, legs bent, feet flat on the floor, knees pointing up to the ceiling and concentrate on your breathing for a few minutes, to give your mind a chance to clear and your body the opportunity to relax and let go of any tensions that it has accumulated throughout the day.

As you progress and develop your strength and ability and move on to more challenging exercises, don't give up the 'easier' versions of exercises entirely. You will find it extremely useful to include these earlier moves, using them as warm-ups for the harder variations.

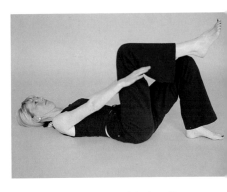

▲ Most people begin to feel the benefits of regular Pilates exercise after only a few sessions.

want to know more?

Take it to the next level...

Go to...
▶ **Posture** – page 27
▶ **The abdominal core** – page 31

Have a go...
▶ **Online anatomy and physiology tutorial** http://www.gwc.maricopa.edu/ home_pages/crimando/jctuts5.htm

Other sources
▶ **Pilates magazines and books** for a wide range of Pilates publications, try your local library and the Internet
▶ **Sports and leisure centre courses** enrol in a Pilates course for beginners at your local sports or leisure centre

getting

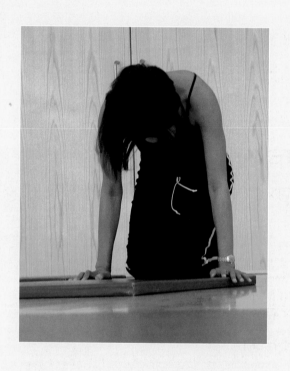

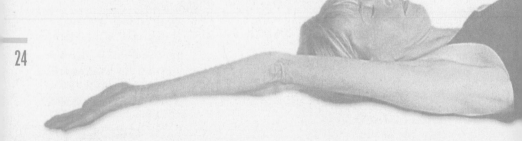

ready

Although Pilates need not be a particularly strenuous form of exercise, it is important to prepare properly in order to gain the maximum benefit from the discipline. Breathing and posture are two of the most important elements of Pilates, as are the basic starting position – the neutral position – and an understanding of the importance of the abdominal core.

Breathing & posture

Good breathing technique and correct posture are central to the successful performance of the Pilates technique. Without these you will not fully benefit from your exercise sessions.

WATCH OUT!

Be prepared
If you suffer from any complaint, are recovering from illness or injury, are pregnant, or have recently lost or gained weight, it is essential that you seek medical advice before committing yourself to any new exercise programme.

Breathing correctly results in an increased efficiency of oxygen supply to the muscles. Many of us have developed the habit of breathing primarily into the chest, raising the ribcage upwards as we inhale. Under the Pilates system, the breathing action is focussed on the lower part of the ribcage and the back. As we breathe in, instead of lifting the ribs upwards, we expand them out to the side and out at the back, breathing deeply to take air to the bottom of the lungs, as far as possible. The chest is not involved in this action and remains as relaxed as possible. This method of breathing is known as 'thoracic' or 'lateral' breathing and, in Pilates, this technique is sometimes referred to as breathing 'full and wide'.

Thoracic breathing

For the correct technique, follow these steps:

1. Stand with your feet in parallel, hip-width apart, your weight centred and evenly distributed over both feet. Place the palms of your hands at the base of your ribs, with the middle fingers of your left and right hands touching slightly. Relax your shoulders and draw your shoulderblades down into your back. Your legs should be straight, but make sure that you are not locking your knees – keep them 'soft' (slightly bent).

2. Breathe in, keeping the chest relaxed and the shoulders down, focus on the lower part of the ribcage. As you inhale, imagine that your

ribcage is expanding out to the sides and out at the back. As your ribcage expands, your fingers and hands will separate slightly. Breathe out, relaxing the ribcage and allowing the hands to return to the starting position. Repeat several times, but avoid overdoing it and hyperventilating. Stop immediately if you start to feel dizzy.

The timing of the breathing is also important in Pilates – whether we breathe in or out as we move can change the quality of the movement itself. The general rule is that we breathe in to prepare, breathe out to move and breathe in to recover.

Co-ordinating the movements of the body with the breathing pattern requires us to establish a rhythm, both in our movement and our breathing. All Pilates movements should be smooth and even and performed in perfect time with the breath.

Posture

Correct posture is essential to Pilates. Most of us have learned various bad habits over the years, causing stress to our bodies and resulting in stiffness, tension and even pain. Pilates offers us the means to re-educate our bodies and correct any weaknesses or bad habits.

In practising Pilates, we focus continually on working with the body in the correct alignment, using the central core to support us as we move. This means that, over time, our posture automatically improves and we begin to find ourselves standing with our spine in good alignment, our shoulders relaxed and our weight evenly spread over both feet. Consequently, no matter what activity we are doing, we will automatically choose a position in which the body can function at its best without risk of strain or injury to any of the muscles or joints.

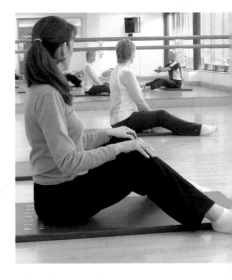

▲ If you have never tried a fitness routine before, you are advised to consider attending classes where you can work under the instruction of an experienced teacher.

The neutral position

Working from what is known as the neutral position, or neutral spine, is one of the key elements in the Pilates method. This is the term used to describe the position of the body when our spine is in its correct alignment.

This is not a precise posture, as each person is different and will therefore have a slightly different natural, or neutral position. However, when correctly aligned, the spine forms a slight 'S'-shape, which is made up of three natural curves – the neck (cervical vertebrae), the upper back (thoracic vertebrae) and the lumbar spine (lumbar vertebrae). Using the Pilates technique,

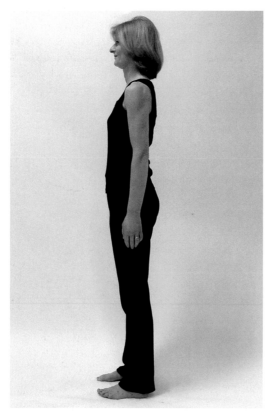

◄ Everyone's neutral position is slightly different, but this is the basic stance – the spine is in its natural position, neither flattened out or over-arched.

it is essential to develop the ability to find and maintain this neutral spine position while standing, sitting, or lying down.

Standing in the neutral position

1. Stand with your feet in parallel, hip-width apart, legs straight and knees soft, shoulders relaxed and down, and arms resting by your sides. Check that your weight is evenly distributed over both feet with your knees positioned directly above your ankles.

2. Make sure that your head is balanced correctly on the top of the spine and that you are not jutting your chin forwards or pulling your head back. Draw the shoulderblades down into your back and keep your shoulders relaxed and down away from your ears, without either pulling them back or rounding them forward.

3. Now imagine that there is a thread running through your spine, with one end coming out of the top of your head and travelling up towards the ceiling, and the other coming out through your tailbone down to the floor. Allow this image to help you lengthen all the way along the spine and neck as you imagine sending the crown of your head up to the ceiling and your tailbone down to the floor.

4. You are now standing in what is known as the neutral position. Your back is neither flattened-out nor arched forwards, but correctly aligned, in a slight 'S' shape, following its natural curves.

5. If you wish, try flattening your back out and then arching it forwards a few times, until you are confident you have found the middle or 'neutral' point.

The feet

As we stand, our body should be centred, with our weight evenly distributed over both feet. It is also important that our weight is correctly focussed on the feet, and that we are not leaning back, forwards, or too much to one side.

- Imagine that there is a triangle on the base of each foot with one side of the triangle running between the big toe and the little toe, and the other two sides running from each of these toes down to the heel. Think of this triangle as your base and concentrate on distributing your weight evenly over this.
- Keep your feet flat on the floor – make sure you do not roll them either inwards or outwards.
- Avoid clenching your toes.

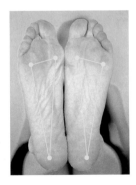

▲ Imagine that there are triangles on the base of your feet – think of your weight being evenly distributed over these two triangles as you stand.

GETTING READY

Sitting in the neutral position

1. Sit on the edge of a chair, with your feet flat on the floor, hip-width apart, your hands either relaxed by your sides or resting on your thighs. Tilt your pelvis forward and round your back, flattening out your lumbar spine and curving the body forward very slightly.

2. Next, tilt your pelvis backward, and arch your lower back.

3. Keep moving between these points until you find the mid position (neutral), with your back straight and a slight natural curve in your lower back.

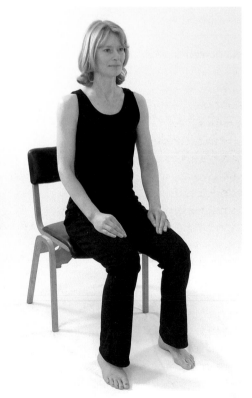

◀ Tilt your pelvis backwards and forwards until you find your neutral position.

Neutral position lying down

1. Lie on your back with your feet hip-width apart, knees pointing up to the ceiling, your arms by your sides, palms facing down.

2. Tilt your pelvis forward, flattening your lower back, raising your tailbone up away from the floor and lifting your ribs.

3. Now arch your lower back, pressing your tailbone down into the floor and lifting the lower spine away from the floor.

4. Move between these two points until you find your neutral position, with your tailbone on the floor and a slight gap between your waist and the floor – just sufficient for you to slide your hand under your lower back (opposite).

5. Once you have found your neutral position your hips should remain level and stable.

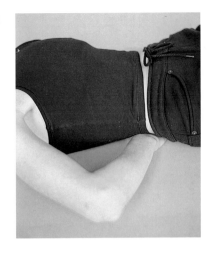

▲ There should be a slight gap – enough for you to slide your hand under your lower back.

The abdominal core

A fundamental factor of Pilates is that all exercises are performed with the support and control of the central (abdominal) core. The aim is to create a strong, stable centre from which we can perform our entire range of movements. Focussing on supporting the movement from our abdominal core, allows us to exercise the body while giving support to the lower back, thereby reducing any risk of stress or strain to the lower spine.

Before we begin any movement, we contract the abdominals. Pull the pelvic floor muscles upwards and inwards (a feeling similar to that of attempting to interrupt the flow of urine) as the abdominal muscles are drawn back towards the lumbar spine. Some refer to this as 'navel to spine' or even 'zip and hollow' (i.e. 'zip' up with the pelvic floor muscles and 'hollow' the abdominals back towards the spine).

want to know more?

Take it to the next level...

Go to...
▶ **Breathing** – page 34
▶ **Physiology** – pages 12–15

Have a go...
▶ **Creative visualization**
before each exercise session, take a minute to create a positive picture of yourself – visualize yourself as a healthy, happy person, bubbling over with energy

Other sources
▶ **Breathing techniques**
search online for breathwork to try out
▶ **Alexander Technique**
an excellent general bodywork system

warm-up

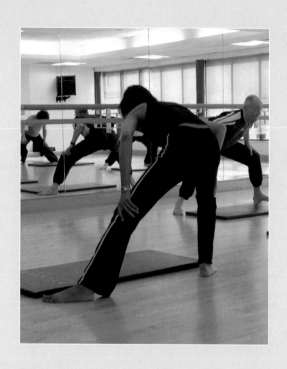

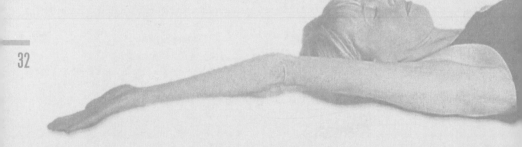

moves

Warming up is an important
element in any exercise
routine and should never be
missed out. It allows you to
gently stretch and mobilize
the body, increasing the
circulation and activating
and warming the muscles
in preparation for the more
intensive exercises ahead.

Breathing

Integral to the success of Pilates, good breathing is an important part of the warm-up procedure. Take your time to get your breathing right before beginning the exercises.

1. Lie on the floor with your knees bent and pointing straight up to the ceiling, feet flat on the floor in parallel. Place your hands on your lower ribs, elbows pointing out to the sides. Drop your shoulders and draw your shoulderblades down into your back. Make sure that your spine is in neutral and your back and neck lengthened.

2. Breathe in, as deeply as you can, into the lower ribs and the back. You should be able to feel the movement of your ribs under your hands as your ribs expand out to the sides, and the slight pressure of your back against the floor as it expands. Breathe out and release.

4. Repeat five to ten times, trying to increase the movement of the ribs each time. Keep the chest relaxed throughout – do not hunch the shoulders or tense the neck as you breathe.

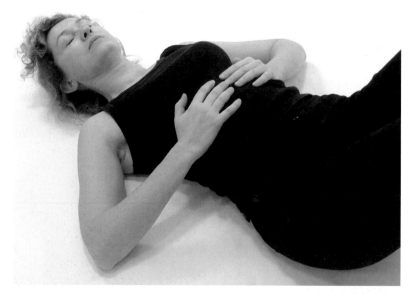

▲ Feel the movement of your ribs as they expand out to the sides when you breathe in and out.

Rolling down the wall

This basic warm-up exercise will assist with regulating breathing and will help you to begin concentrating on the abdominal core, which is central to all Pilates technique.

1. Stand with your back against a wall or door, feet in parallel, hip-width apart, heels approximately 30–45cm (12–18in) away from the wall. Drop your shoulders and let your arms hang relaxed by your sides.

2. Bend your knees slightly, tucking your pelvis under and take a deep breath. Exhale slowly, contract your abdominals, bend your head forwards, and slowly begin to roll down through the spine, peeling your spine away from the wall vertebra by vertebra, directing the top of your head down towards the floor. Keep your knees bent and your arms and hands relaxed. If you run out of breath pause, take another breath, and continue rolling all the way down to the floor, increasing the bend in your knees, if necessary.

3. Breathe in, contract the abdominals and start to roll slowly back up through the spine, vertebra by vertebra, again taking an extra breath as you go if necessary. Keep your head bent forwards until the last moment, as you straighten up. Repeat five times.

▼ Roll down the wall gradually, concentrating on moving one vertebra at a time as you lower.

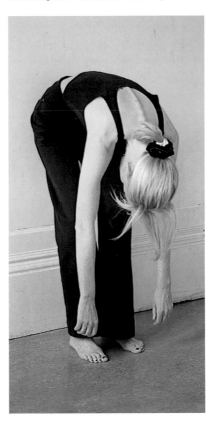

Standing balance

Maintaining good balance is an important part of most Pilates exercises, so it is as well to concentrate on finding your bodily equilibrium as you warm up in preparation.

1. Stand with your feet slightly apart, knees soft, spine in neutral. Lengthen along the spine and back of the neck. Drop your shoulders, draw your shoulderblades right back and down behind you and relax the arms. Focus your eyes straight ahead and breathe in.

2. Breathe out slowly, contract the abdominal muscles, and continue lengthening up through the spine, allowing your heels to raise up away from the ground. Imagine the top of your head lifting straight up towards the ceiling while at the same time your tailbone releases down to the floor. Remember to keep your eyes directed straight ahead, as this will help you to maintain your balance.

3. Keep rolling up through your feet as you breathe out, until you are balanced on your toes. Do not let your ankles bend out to the sides as you raise up.

4. When you have raised up as far as possible, breathe in, lengthening up through the spine as much as you possibly can.

5. Breathe out, contract the abdominals and slowly lower yourself back down, continuing to lengthen up through the spine as you do so. Repeat the exercise five to ten times.

▶ To help your balance, choose a point directly in front of you and keep your eyes focussed on this point as you roll up and down through your feet.

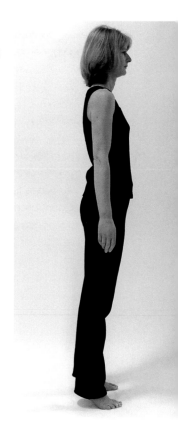

Arm swings

**The purpose of arm swings as part
of the general Pilates warm-up is to
loosen the muscles of the arms,
shoulders and upper torso. Synchronize
your breathing with the arm swings.**

1. Stand with your feet in parallel, hip-width apart,
   and your spine in neutral. Lengthen along the
   spine and neck, breathe in and raise your
   arms up towards the ceiling, directing them
   away from the body very slightly. Keep your
   shoulders dropped and your shoulderblades
   pulled down into your back.

2. Breathe out, contract the abdominal muscles
   and swing your arms downwards and then
   back behind you, bending your knees,
   relaxing your head and shoulders, bending
   your head forwards and curving the spine
   over as you do so.

3. Breathe in and slowly swing the arms back
   and roll back up to the starting position.
   Repeat the swings five to ten times in a
   continous, controlled, smooth movement,
   lengthening the spine up towards the ceiling
   a little more each time as you roll back up
   to standing.

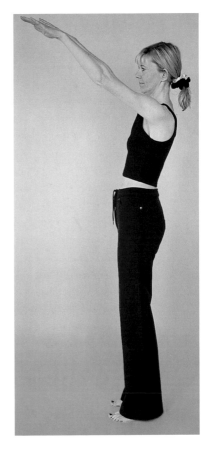

▲ Keep your shoulders dropped
down away from your ears as you
swing your arms.

Arm raises into arm circles

A more advanced version of arm swings, this exercise continues the process of working all your arm and upper body muscle groups.

1. Stand with your feet in parallel, slightly apart. Place your left hand on your right rib cage to make sure that you do not raise your ribs up as you lift your arm. Breathe in and raise your right arm in front of you, slightly to the side.

2. Breathe in and raise your right arm up, floating the right hand up towards the ceiling. Lengthen the arm out of the shoulder joint as you lift. Keep your shoulder dropped and your ribs soft.

3. Breathe out and slowly lower your arm. Repeat the sequence five times.

4. Breathe in and raise your right arm as before; as you breathe out, take the arm over and back to the starting position, in a circular motion. Keep your shoulder down.

5. Repeat five times, keeping the circles even, in time with the breathing; reverse the direction for five more circles. Repeat for the left arm.

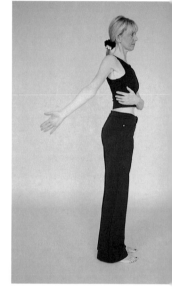

▲ Start by working each arm individually, resting the opposite hand on your ribs to check that you are not lifting the ribs and you circle the arms.

Option

1. Repeat the sequence once more, this time using both arms together.

2. Raise and lower the arms five times, then circle the arms five times in each direction, breathing in as you circle the arms up and breathing out as you circle them back down to the starting position. You will find that when circling both arms together you will probably need to make the circles smaller to keep your shoulders dropped throughout the move.

Shoulder hunches

The shoulders can harbour a great deal of muscular tension. One good way to alleviate any stiffness and prepare the muscles for exercise is to warm up with shoulder hunches.

1. Stand with your feet in parallel, hip-width apart, arms by your sides, with your spine in neutral.

2. Breathe in to a count of two and hunch both your shoulders up to your ears, as high as you can. Keep your arms as relaxed as possible, and your spine and neck in neutral throughout.

3. Breathe out to a count of four as you slowly drop your shoulders back down away from your ears.

4. Repeat the entire sequence five times, trying to drop your shoulders even further down a little more each time as you complete the exercise.

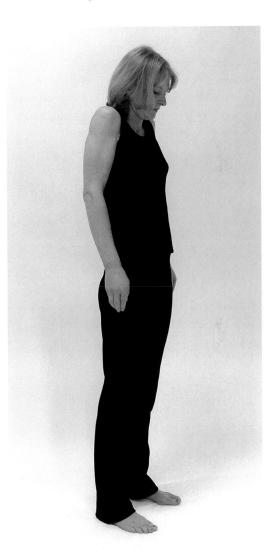

▲ Shrug your shoulders, then drop them as far as possible to get the most benefit from this simple but effective move.

▶ Alternate hip openings

**This warm-up exercise opens up the pelvis, hip joints
and groin, loosening them up and preparing them for the
more strenuous exercise ahead.**

1. Lie on your back with your feet in parallel,
   hip-width apart, your spine in neutral. Place
   your hands palms down on your abdomen,
   fingertips on your pubic bone and your
   thumbs touching, to form a triangle. As you

▼ Forming the 'pelvic
triangle' with the hands.

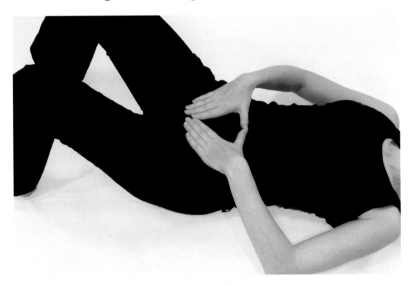

WATCH OUT!

Stretch slowly

Embark on this exercise slowly and carefully, as it is
relatively easy to sustain groin or hip strain if you
push your legs outwards too hard or too quickly. If
you are of advanced age, have osteoporosis or
have recently had a hip replacement, consult your
doctor before attempting this exercise.

drop each knee out to the side, the area under your hands should stay completely level. Breathe in.

2. Breathe out, contract the abdominals and, keeping your foot in position, slowly let your right knee drop out to the side a little, opening out the hip joint. As you drop the knee, check that your tailbone does not tilt up, and make sure that your hips stay level, with both buttocks in contact with the floor: if your left hip starts to raise up, then you are dropping the right knee too far. Your left leg should remain stable throughout, with your left knee pointing up towards the ceiling.

3. Breathe in as you return the knee back to the starting position. Repeat five times on the right side then change legs and repeat five times on the left.

▼ This exercise mobilizes the hip joints, opens up the pelvic area and releases tension in the lower back.

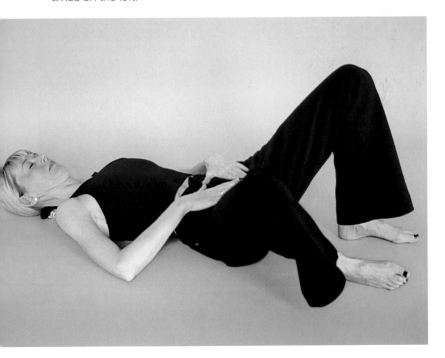

Hip folds

Just as arm swings and arm raises into arm circles will prepare your arms and upper torso for the later exercises, hip folds stimulate and stretch the leg muscles and pelvis.

1. Lie on your back with your feet in parallel, hip-width apart, knees bent and pointing up to the ceiling, your spine in neutral and your arms by your sides. Breathe in.

2. Breathe out, contract your abdominals and float your right knee up until the knee is at a right angle, with the shin parallel to the floor.

3. Breathe in, holding this position, then breathe out as you lower your foot back down to the floor. Repeat ten times, alternating the legs each time.

Option 1

1. Breathe out as you contract the abdominal muscles and float the right knee up as above. Breathe in, then breathe out and float the left leg up to join it.

▼ Option 1: Make sure that you keep your abdominals contracted and your spine in neutral as you 'dip' each foot in turn down towards the floor.

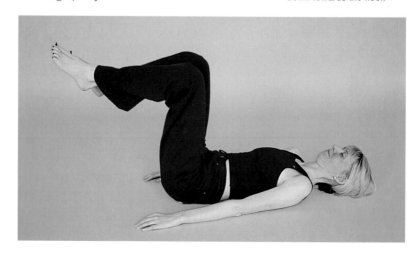

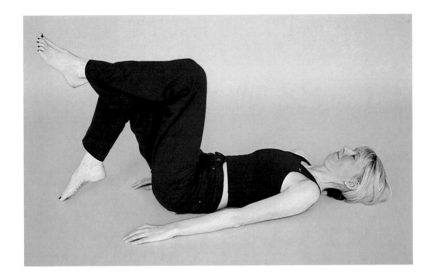

2. Breathe out and lower the right foot to the floor, breathe in, then breathe out and lower the left foot.

3. Repeat the sequence, this time raising the left leg first. Repeat the entire sequence six to ten times.

▲ Option 2: Again, ensure that you hold your neutral spine position and keep your abdominals contracted as you complete the deep toe dips in this version of the exercise.

Option 2

1. Breathe out as you contract the abdominal muscles and float the right knee up as above. Breathe in, then breathe out and float the left leg up to join it.

2. Breathe out, then, using a continuous movement, lower the right foot towards the floor, toes softly pointed, and very gently touch the toes of your right foot onto the floor (as if you were dipping your toes into a pool of water). Raise your leg back up to join the right. Repeat for the left leg.

3. Repeat the toe dips five times on each leg, alternating the legs each time.

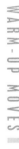

Egyptian arm circles

This is one of the most complete upper body warm-up exercises you can undertake before you embark on a Pilates routine. The lower body should stay relaxed throughout.

1. Lie on your back with your knees bent, feet flat on the floor in parallel, hip-width apart, arms by your sides, palms down. Check your spine is in neutral.

2. Breathe out, contract the abdominals and float your hands up towards the ceiling, until they are level with your shoulders, keeping your arms straight and your elbows soft. Breathe in.

3. Breathe out, bend your elbows so that they are at right angles and bring your upper arms down to the floor, in line with your

▼ Float your hands up towards the ceiling, keeping your arms straight and your elbows soft.

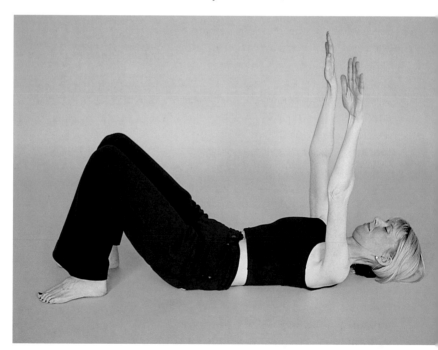

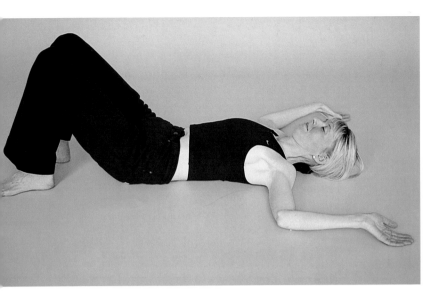

shoulders, forearms and hands still pointing up towards the ceiling.

4. Breathe in and bring your forearms down to the floor, so that they lie either side of the head, palms facing upwards, elbows at right angles.

5. Breathe out as you continue the movement, straightening your elbows as you lengthen the arms away from you along the ground until they are in parallel, hands shoulder-width apart. Then float them up to the ceiling, keeping the elbows straight, until the arms are back in the starting position, with the arms at shoulder level, fingers pointing straight up to the ceiling. Breathe in.

6. Repeat five times, then repeat five times in the opposite direction. Breathe out as you take the arms above the head and down to the floor, breathe in as you bend the elbows, breathe out as you lift the hands and forearms, then straighten the arms, taking your hands straight up towards the ceiling.

▲ Keep your knees parallel, pointing straight up at the ceiling as you move the arms.

want to know **more?**

Take it to the next level...

Go to...
▶ **Principles of Pilates** – pages 16–17
▶ **Warm-ups** – pages 164–7

Have a go...
▶ **Improve your concentration**
  with some simple and highly effective exercises – visit www.braingym.org
▶ **Monitor your progress**
  start a Pilates journal to help you quickly and easily see the progress you are making and keep you motivated

Other sources
▶ **Websites on 'why warm up?'**
  check out websites devoted to warm-ups

stand

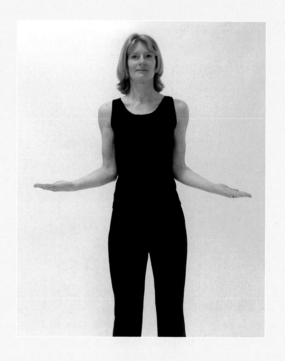

up

The Pilates technique involves a series of exercises designed to improve all aspects of mind and body harmony, while working the different muscle groups and parts of the body. The exercises that are performed standing up primarily work the spine, arms and torso.

Rolling down

This is a great exercise for strengthening the spine and improving flexibility. Keep your abdominals contracted and your knees 'soft' (slightly bent) to support your lower back.

1. Stand in neutral with your feet hip-width apart, your knees soft (slightly bent) and your weight evenly balanced over both feet. Lengthen through the spine, thinking of sending the crown of your head up to the ceiling and your tailbone down to the floor. Breathe in and contract your lower abdominals.

2. Breathe out, drop your chin onto your chest and start to roll slowly down through the spine, letting the weight of your head draw you down towards the floor. Keep your arms relaxed and your knees soft and avoid sticking the tailbone out – keep thinking of sending it down to the floor.

3. Roll down at a slow, even pace: if you run out of breath, pause and inhale, then exhale and continue rolling the rest of the way down to the floor. Think of curling down through the spine one vertebra at a time, starting at the top and working all the way down to the tailbone.

WATCH OUT!

Watch your back
If you have a back or neck problem or injury of any kind, seek medical advice before attempting this move, as it puts quite a lot of pressure on the spine.

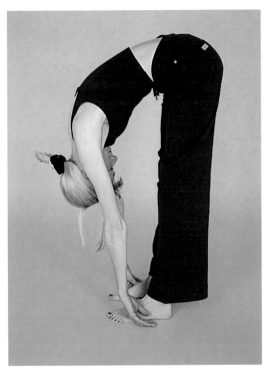

◄ As you roll down towards the floor, check that your neck and arms are completely relaxed. If your hamstrings are tight or stiff, then allow your knees to bend as you roll down – this exercise is intended to mobilize the spine and not necessarily to stretch the leg muscles.

4. When you have gone as far as you are comfortably able, breathe in, contract the abdominals and breathe out as you reverse the process and slowly roll back up through the spine, to a standing position. Leave your head dropped forwards until the last moment. Again, if you run out of breath, pause and inhale, then exhale and continue to roll back up to standing.

MUST KNOW

Benefits
- Strengthens the abdominals and the spine.
- Increases flexibility in the back.
- Releases tension in the back and shoulders.

Arm raises

When you perform these arm raises, keep the spine fully lengthened and the body facing forwards. Avoid leaning to one side or swaying backwards or forwards as you lift the arms.

1. Stand with your feet hip-width apart and your spine in neutral, arms relaxed by your sides.

2. Breathe in as you lengthen through the spine and neck, relax and drop your shoulders drawing the shoulderblades down into your back.

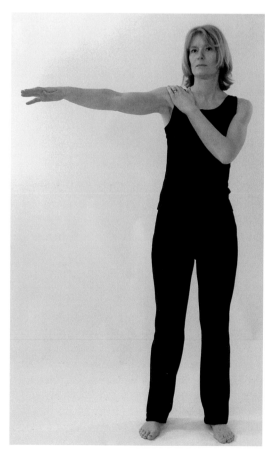

◄ Keep your outstretched hand as relaxed as possible throughout the move.

MUST KNOW

Benefits
- Improves posture.
- Strengthens the arm and shoulder muscles.
- Relieves tension in the neck and shoulders.
- Improves breath control.

3. Breathe out and slowly raise your right arm out to the side up to shoulder level, lengthening it away from you, keeping the elbow soft and the outstretched hand relaxed, palm facing down. Keep the shoulders dropped down, away from your ears, and the shoulderblades drawn back and down behind you as much as possible as you lift.

4. When your arm is at shoulder level, rotate your arm so that the palm faces up towards the ceiling.

5. Breathe in as you rotate the hand back and then gradually lower your arm. Repeat three to five times.

6. Repeat for the other side. Then repeat the sequence once more, raising both arms at the same time.

WATCH OUT!

Remain comfortable

If you find it difficult to lift the arms to shoulder level while keeping the body in the correct position, then take them lower until your strength and muscle control improves sufficiently for you to raise them comfortably to shoulder height. If you are unsure whether you are lifting your arm too high, place your other hand on your shoulder so you can feel if you are raising it above shoulder level.

STAND UP

51

Waist twist (Cossack arms)

This movement is primarily a spine rotation, so take it gently and focus on correcting any imbalances until you can achieve a smooth and controlled movement.

WATCH OUT!

- Do not twist round too far – rotate from the waist, keeping the head in line with the body.
- If you suffer from back or neck problems, seek medical advice before attempting this exercise.

1. Stand with your legs hip-width apart, feet in parallel. Drop your shoulders and pull your shoulderblades down into your back. Lengthen up through the spine and back of the neck.

2. Breathe in and bring your arms up to just below shoulder level, placing one forearm on top of the other, with the fingers of one hand touching the elbow of the opposite arm, in a 'Cossack'-style pose as illustrated on the opposite page. Do not hunch the shoulders as you bring the arms up.

3. Breathe out, lengthen up out of the waist and slowly twist round to the right with the upper body, making sure that you keep your hips facing forwards. Avoid rounding the shoulders forward or leaning back as you twist round and release the back. Keep the head in line with the shoulders – do not be tempted to take it any further round than the rest of the body. When you reach your

MUST KNOW

Benefits
- Stretches the waist and upper back.
- Improves the posture.
- Releases tension in the spine.

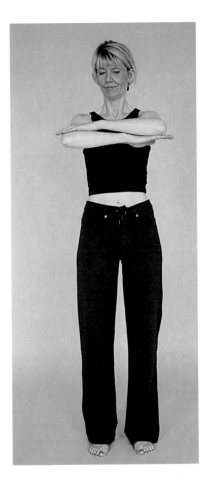

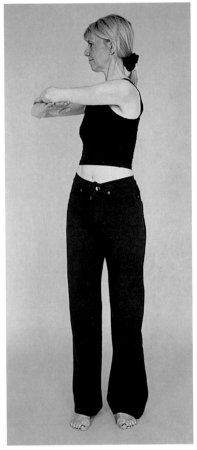

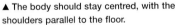
▲ The body should stay centred, with the shoulders parallel to the floor.

▲ Keep the shoulders dropped and the shoulderblades drawn down into the back.

tension point, try to relax your body a little more, using your breathing, while still maintaining your posture. Twist round as far as you can, keeping the movement slow and controlled, then breathe in and return to centre. Keep your hips facing forward as you twist – the actual twisting movement occurs in the upper body only, not from the hips. Repeat the move for the other side. Repeat the sequence five to ten times, trying to increase the twist gradually each time.

▶ Chest opener

This movement emphasizes mobility and is a great warm-up for your chest muscles. It will also help you develop better all-round posture.

1. Stand with your back in neutral and your feet in parallel, hip-width apart. Your spine and neck should be lengthened and your arms resting by your sides. Your legs should be straight with your knees soft. Tuck your elbows into your waist, and raise your hands up to waist level, palms facing upwards. Focus your eyes straight ahead in front of you.

▼ Make sure that you keep your shoulders down and your elbows tucked in to your waist throughout this exercise.

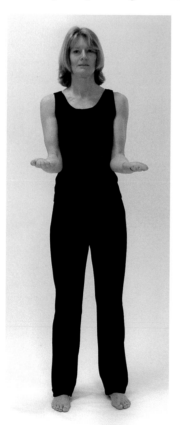

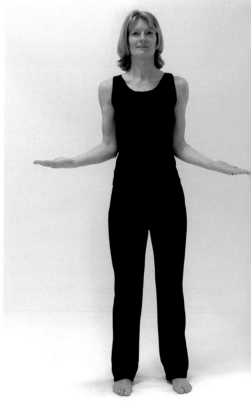

▶ Keep the movement slow and smooth as you return your hands to the centre, with the elbows remaining at a 90-degree angle.

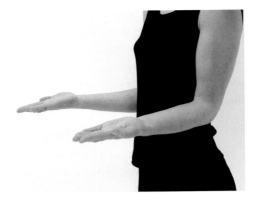

2. Breathe out, contracting the abdominals, dropping the shoulders and drawing the shoulderblades down into your back, remaining as relaxed as possible, trying to release any tension from your neck and shoulders.

3. Breathe in and take your hands slowly out to the sides and back as far as possible. Keep dropping your shoulders and drawing your shoulderblades down and back as you do this. Breathe out and slowly bring your hands back to centre. Keep the movement slow and smooth. Your speed should be constant. Repeat five to ten times, moving the hands at an even pace, in time with the breath.

Option

This exercise can be done either sitting or standing. If you wish to sit, position yourself forward on the chair and place your feet hip-width apart on the floor in front of you. Make sure that your spine is in neutral, with your back and neck lengthened.

MUST KNOW

Benefits

- Improves posture.
- Works the upper arms and shoulders.
- Releases tension at the base of the neck and across the tops of the shoulders.
- Opens the chest.

Push up

This is a flowing movement that should be performed slowly and evenly, using a controlled movement. Remember to keep your abdominals contracted and breathe evenly.

1. Stand with feet hip-width apart and knees soft, weight evenly distributed over both feet. Breathe in and contract your lower abdominals.

2. Breathe out, drop your head forward and start to roll down through the spine, vertebra by vertebra, using a slow, controlled movement.

3. Continue to roll down as you exhale, pausing to take an extra breath if you need to, resting your hands lightly on your knees.

MUST KNOW

Benefits
• Strengthens the abdominals, the lower back, the upper body and the arms.

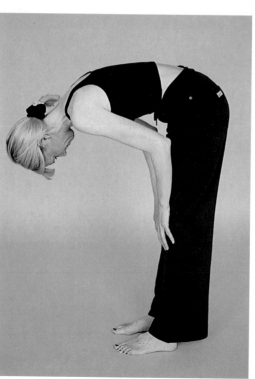

◄ As you roll down through the spine, allow your hands to come to rest lightly on your knees.

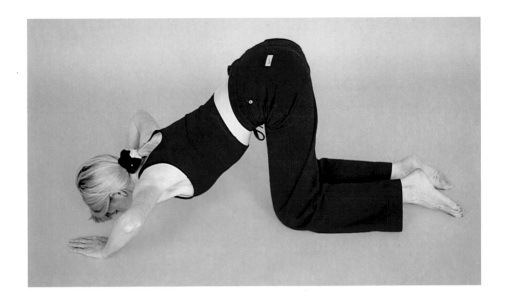

4. When you have gone as far as you are comfortably able, bend your knees and place your hands onto the floor, fingertips first. Focus your eyes straight down at the floor and keep lengthening through the neck. Breathe in, then breathe out and walk your hands forward away from your body, gently dropping to your knees as you do so, until you are on all fours, with your knees directly below your hips and your hands directly below your shoulders.

5. Breathe in and, using a slow, even movement, breathe out and lower your upper body down the floor, sending your elbows out away from the body, and then push back up. Keep your abdominals contracted and your hips level. Repeat this push up five to ten times, exhaling as you lower and inhaling as you rise. To finish, breathe in, then breathe out as you walk your hands back, take your weight onto your feet and slowly roll back up to standing, bringing your head up last.

▲ Keep your lower abdominals contracted to focus the strengthening effect of the move and support your lower back.

want to know more?

Take it to the next level...

Go to...
▶ **The neutral position** – page 29
▶ **The legs** – page 174

Have a go...
▶ **Staying active**
as possible all day long will help your fitness
▶ **Cardiovascular exercise**
should be included in your weekly exercise routine. Do aerobics, go for a run or simply take a brisk walk

Other sources
▶ **Fitness websites**
such as www.worldfitness.com offer information on general fitness, Pilates, yoga, nutrition and much more

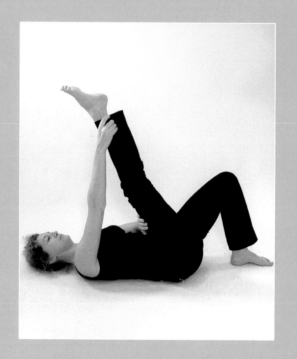

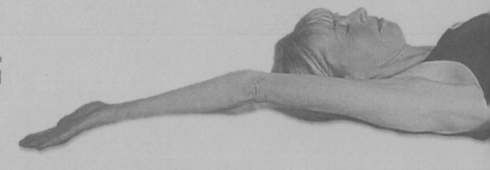

down

The Pilates method was first developed as a set of rehabilitation exercises for patients. However, this does not mean that Pilates is in any way a soft option. The exercises that are performed lying down allow each of the muscle groups to be worked on in turn, while also supporting the spine.

▶ Spine curls

By working on this exercise, you will find that not only will your back become more supple and flexible, but that your stomach muscles will become stronger and more toned.

1. Lie on your back with feet hip-width apart, knees bent, feet flat on the floor, heels as close to your body as possible, and arms resting by your sides. Lengthen through the spine and along the back of the neck.

2. Breathing out, contract the abdominals and tilt the pelvis up slightly, keeping the spine in contact with the floor. Breathe in and release, then breathe out, tilt the pelvis raising it slightly off the floor. Repeat, lifting the tailbone off the floor a little more each time, gradually peeling the spine away the floor, vertebra by vertebra. Breathe out as you lift and breathe in as you release the spine back down to the floor.

▼ Keep the hips level, in line with the shoulders, and the knees stable throughout this exercise.

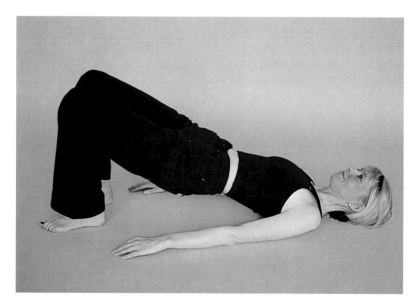

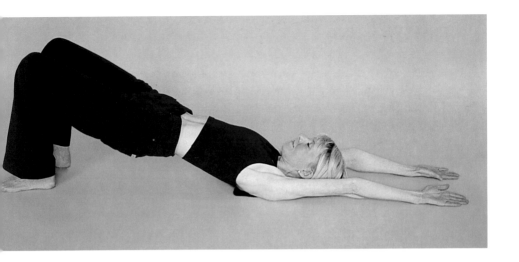

3. Breathe out, contract the abdominals and roll the tailbone up off the floor until you are resting on your shoulders, with the body in a diagonal slope, keeping the spine in neutral. Breathe in. Breathe out as you contract the abdominals and roll the spine slowly back down to the starting position. Repeat three to five times.

4. Repeat step 3, but now, once you reach the diagonal position, breathe in and slowly raise the arms up over the head and down to the floor, then breathe out as you bring them back to the starting position. Breathe in, then breathe out as you roll down through the spine onto the floor.

▲ Use a smooth, controlled movement as you slowly peel the spine away from the floor then roll back down again.

Option

Keep the arms in position over your head as you breathe out and roll back down through the spine, then breathe in as you bring the arms back. Repeat the move five to ten times.

MUST KNOW

Benefits
• Increases flexibility in the spine.
• Strengthens muscles in abdominal and pelvic areas.
• Improves muscle control.

▶ Arm circles

This is a great exercise for improving arm and shoulder strength, while at the same time releasing any tension that you hold in your chest, shoulders and neck.

1. Lie on your back with your legs bent, ankles hip-width apart, feet flat on the floor. Place your arms by your sides. Drop the shoulders, drawing the shoulderblades into your back. Check that the spine is in neutral. Breathe in, contracting the abdominals and bring the arms up to shoulder level, holding the hands shoulder-width apart, pointing straight up to the ceiling, palms facing away from you, towards your feet.

2. Breathe out, making small, slow circles with your arms, taking the arms up towards the head, around and out, then down and back up to the starting position. Breathe out as you take the arms up and away from the body, inhale as you bring them down and back in. Repeat five times

▼ Maintain the spine in the neutral position and the abdominals contracted throughout this sequence.

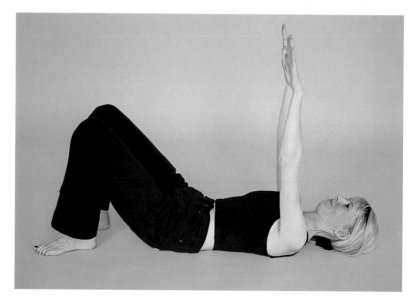

Benefits

- Strengthens the abdominal muscles.
- Gently stretches and strengthens the arms.
- Releases tension in the shoulders and chest.

using an even motion. Keep the arms and shoulders as relaxed as possible, elbows soft, with the shoulderblades drawn into your back.

3. Repeat, changing the direction of the arm circles, exhaling as you take the hands down towards the body and out, then inhaling as you bring them up and round. Repeat five times. Change direction again and repeat the sequence one more time, making five circles in one direction, then five in the other. Once you are familiar with this exercise you can gradually make the circles bigger. If you have any tension in the shoulders, try sliding the arms along the floor as you bring the arms down and round.

▼ Repeat the exercise, changing the direction of the arm rotations and focussing on your breathing.

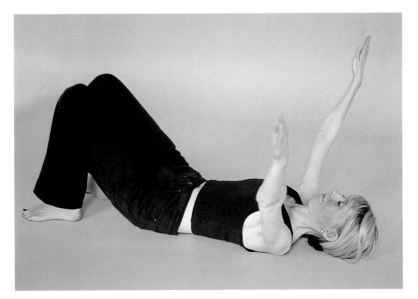

LYING DOWN

▶ Hip rolls

With this particular exercise, use your abdominals to control the move as you roll. Do not simply allow the weight of the legs to pull you over to the floor.

1. Lie on your back in neutral, your legs bent, knees hip-width apart and pointing up to the ceiling, feet in parallel. Place your arms out to the sides with palms facing upwards. Breathe in and lengthen along the spine and back of the neck and relax the body, allowing the floor to support your weight.

2. Breathe out, contract the abdominals and let your knees roll gently over to one side very

▼ As you rotate the hips in one direction and the head in the other, make sure you keep both shoulders in contact with the floor at all times.

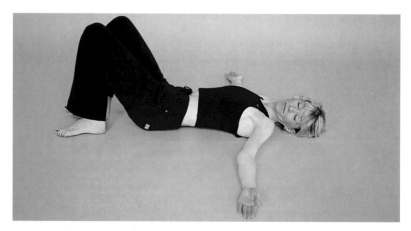

WATCH OUT!

Don't force this stretch – gradually increase the rotation each time, only taking it as far as is comfortable for you. As you develop flexibility in the spine and strength in the abdominal core you will automatically find you will gradually be able to take the stretch further.

slightly (the knees should move just a few inches to start with). At the same time rotate the head in the opposite direction.

3. Breathe in, contract the abdominals and breathe out as you bring the knees back to the starting position. Repeat on the other side.

4. Repeat the sequence five to ten times, taking the knees a little further over each time. As you start to rotate the hips further, allow the hip to lift up as you peel the lower back away from the floor vertebra by vertebra. As you bring the knees back to centre, let the spine roll slowly back down one vertebra at a time.

Option

Once you have developed strength and control in the abdominal core, you can try doing this exercise using the following position.

1. Float your legs up, one at a time, until they are at right angles with the body (knees bent and shins parallel to the floor).

2. Place a tennis ball or small cushion between your knees, to help stabilize the legs, then rotate the hips and the head as above.

MUST KNOW

Benefits
- Stretches the spine and waist muscles.
- Relieves tightness and stiffness in the lower back.
- Gently stretches the neck and releases tension.

▼ Try to keep your knees at right angles, with your shins parallel to the floor and your knees in line with your hips as you slowly roll from side to side.

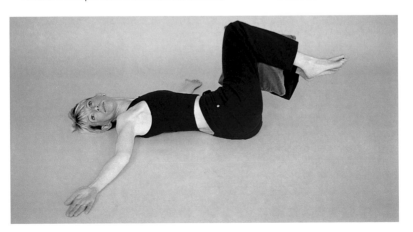

▶ The Hundred

This is a relatively challenging exercise which offers a number of different options. Do not attempt the later options until you have properly mastered the easier levels.

1. Lie on the floor with your legs bent, knees pointing up to the ceiling, feet parallel, and your arms by your sides with palms facing downwards.

2. Check that your spine is in neutral, with your hips level and your eyes focussed up to the ceiling. Breathe in, then, as you breathe out, contract your abdominals and float your right leg up until the shin is parallel to the floor, with the knee at right angles.

3. Holding the leg in this position and keeping the hips stable, drop the shoulders and lengthen the arms, lifting and lowering them in a fairly fast pumping action, five times for each breath in and five times for each breath out. Once you have reached 50 arm pumps, change legs and repeat for the other side.

Option 1

If you already have good strength in your abdominal muscles, you can try this option. As you breathe out, extend the leg, lowering it slightly. Think of lengthening away from the hip, down the leg and out through the foot. Check that your spine is still in neutral with your abdominals contracted slightly. Holding this position, pump the arms as described above.

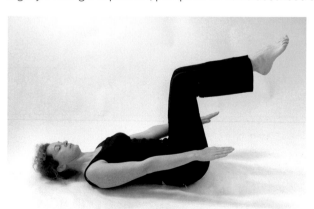

◀ In Option 3, both legs are raised, shins parallel to the floor and knees at right angles for a more challenging exercise.

Option 2

This option increases the intensity of the exercise in the abdominal area. Breathe out and lower the extended leg a little closer to the floor. Holding this position, pump the arms as described above.

Option 3

Adopt the position described in step 1, then breathe in and release your lower back into the floor (this is sometimes referred to as 'imprinting'). Breathe out as you contract your lower abdominals floating your legs up, one after the other, until the shins are parallel to the floor, with the knees at right angles. Pump the arms as described above.

MUST KNOW

There are several developments to this exercise, at various levels of difficulty. Choose an option that suits your current strength and ability. Remember, you will gain far more by working at a less demanding option while maintaining control and alignment, than by struggling with an exercise that is too difficult for you.

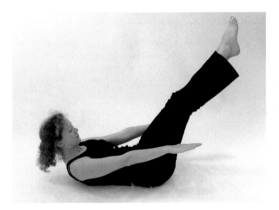

◀ Option 4 is the most difficult move, as the legs are extended and your head and shoulders are raised off the floor. To increase the difficulty, lower the extended legs down towards the floor and hold this position as you pulse with the hands.

Option 4

This is the most difficult option. Follow the instructions for Option 3 then, once you have raised both legs to the right-angle position, breathe in and breathe out, squeeze the inner thighs together. Extend both legs and lower them down towards the floor. At the same time drop your chin to your chest and raise your head off the ground. Pump the arms, as before. Breathe in as you return the legs to the right-angle position, then lower them to the floor, one at a time.

▶ Neck pull

Practising this exercise will help release tension and greatly improve the strength and flexibility of the muscles around the neck, shoulders and upper back.

1. Lie on your back with your spine in neutral and your legs slightly apart, knees bent. Place your hands behind your head, point your elbows out away from the body. Drop your shoulders and draw your shoulderblades down into your back.

WATCH OUT!

If you suffer from any neck problems, seek medical advice before attempting this exercise.

▼ Keep the abdominals contracted to avoid any pressure or strain on the lower back, and make sure that your hands are resting lightly on the back of your head and not pulling on the back of the head as you roll up.

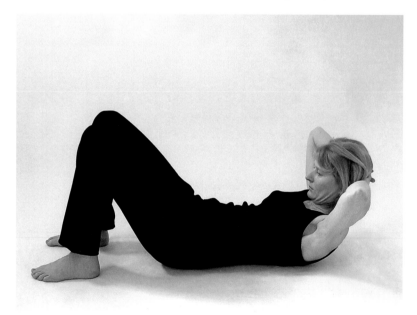

MUST KNOW

Benefits
- Strengthens the abdominal muscles.
- Stretches the neck, shoulders and upper back.
- Increases the flexibility of the spine.

2. Breathe in, lengthen your neck and drop your chin onto your chest very slightly. Breathe out as you contract the abdominals, then slowly raise your head and begin rolling up through the spine. Curl your shoulders away from the floor, vertebra by vertebra, keeping your shoulders down. When you begin to feel resistance in the abdominals, pause, breathe in, then breathe out, increasing the contraction in the abdominals, tilt the pelvis forward, and slowly roll back down to the starting position. Repeat five to ten times.

Option

1. When you have developed sufficient strength in the abdominal core, as well as flexibility in the spine, try repeating the move with your legs extended, knees and ankles together.

2. Roll up through the spine until you reach a sitting position. Continue the movement, breathing in, contracting the abdominals, then breathing out, and curling forward as far as you can.

3. As you stretch forward, imagine rounding your upper body up and over a large beach ball. Inhale and roll back down to the floor. Repeat five to ten times.

▶ Neck stretch

This should be a smooth, slow, gentle stretch of the neck muscles – avoid making any jerky movements or forcing the stretch too far.

1. Lie on the floor with your back in the neutral position, your legs bent, keeping your knees hip-width apart and pointing up to the ceiling, feet in parallel. Place your arms down by your sides with palms down.

2. Breathe in, relax and soften through the chest area, lengthen along the spine and back of the neck, and allow the weight of your body to sink into the floor. Let this happen naturally – do not force the position.

WATCH OUT!

If you experience any pain or discomfort, stop immediately and seek medical advice.

▼ Keep your head on the floor as you move, aiming to roll each ear down to the floor as you roll your head from side to side.

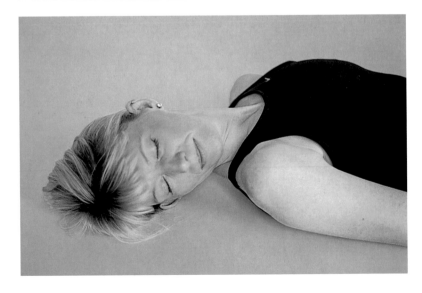

Benefits
- Releases tension and stiffness in the neck.
- Stretches the neck muscles.
- Improves posture.
- Eases neck and shoulder pain.

3. Breathe out and contract the abdominal muscles very slightly then allow your head to roll slowly over to one side, keeping the neck lengthened and the head in contact with the floor. Concentrate on rotating the head and taking the ear towards the floor. Breathe in and bring the head slowly back to centre, then exhale as you roll the head to the other side. Repeat the sequence five to ten times.

4. Starting from the centre position, breathe out and begin to tuck the chin towards the chest, lengthening and stretching the neck. Breathe in as you gently release the chin back up to centre position. Repeat five to ten times.

▼ Keep your shoulders relaxed and your jaw released – make sure you are not clenching your teeth.

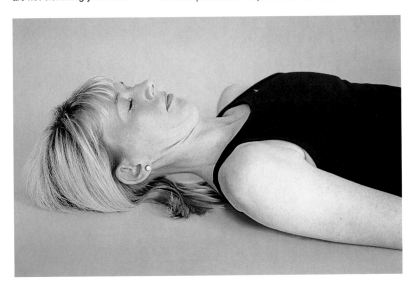

▶ Single leg stretch

This exercise demands concentration to ensure that the hips maintain a stable position, the abdominals are contracted and, when the leg is raised, the knee is at right angles.

1. Lie on your back with your legs bent, knees pointing up to the ceiling, feet in parallel. Place your arms by your sides with palms down.

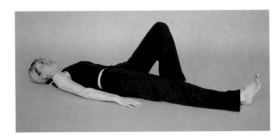

2. Keeping your spine in neutral and your hips stable, in line with your shoulders, breathe in, contract the abdominals, then exhale and extend the right leg, sliding your heel along the ground. Inhale as you slide your leg back to the starting position. Repeat for the left leg. Alternating the legs, repeat 10 to 20 times.

▲ As you exhale, extend your right leg by lengthening the leg away from you, sliding your heel along the floor.

Option 1

1. Once you can confidently extend the legs while keeping the abdominals contracted, the spine in neutral and the hips level, you are ready to try floating the left leg up until the shin is parallel to the floor, knee at right angles. Hold the leg in this position and extend the right leg out, as described in step 1.

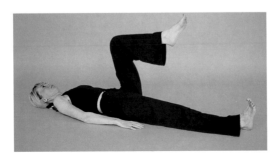

◀ Float the left leg up, making sure the raised knee is kept at right angles and the hips stable.

2. Breathe in and draw the extended leg back to the starting position, then exhale as you float the raised leg back down to the ground. Repeat for the other side. Repeat five to ten times on each side.

▼ Option 2 (left) and Option 3 (right) are further stages of the single leg stretch that can increase the overall intensity of the exercise.

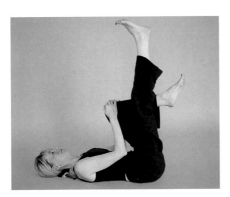 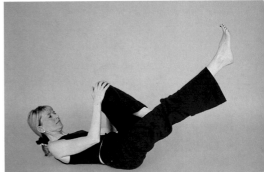

Option 2

1. Float both legs up to towards your chest, one at a time, knees bent. Rest your hands on the outside of your knees, elbows pointing out.

2. Breathe in, contract the abdominals, then breathe out and extend the right leg to the ceiling, placing both hands either side of your left knee as you do so. Breathe in as you bring your right leg back in to your chest. Repeat five to ten times, using alternating legs.

Option 3

1. As the strength in your abdominal muscles increases, try bringing the extended leg closer to the floor to intensify the effect on the abdominal core. Float both legs up towards your chest, one at a time, knees bent. Rest your hands on the outside of your knees, elbows pointing outwards. Drop your chin to your chest slightly, and raise your head away from the floor, lengthening through the neck. Keep your shoulders down and away from your ears, and your shoulderblades pulled down into your back.

2. Breathe in and contract the abdominals, then breathe out and extend the right leg out, placing both hands either side of your left knee. Breathe in as you bring your right leg back in to your chest. Breathe out as you extend the left leg, placing your hands on your right knee. Repeat the sequence five to ten times, keeping the head up throughout.

▶ Double leg stretch

You will find that the arms and abdominal core are strengthened by practising this move, as well as releasing tension in the shoulders and upper body.

1. Lie on your back with legs bent, ankles hip-width apart and feet flat on the floor. Place your arms by your sides. Drop the shoulders, drawing the shoulderblades down into your back. Check that the spine is in neutral. Breathe in and contract the abdominals. Keeping the spine in neutral, bring the arms straight up to shoulder level, holding the hands shoulder-width apart, fingers pointing straight to the ceiling, palms facing away from you towards your feet.

2. Breathe out and float the legs up, one at a time, until the shins are parallel to the floor, with the knees at right angles. Holding the legs in this position, breathe in, then breathe

MUST KNOW

Benefits
- Strengthens the abdominal muscles.
- Gently stretches and strengthens the arms.
- Releases tension in the shoulders and chest.

▼ Maintain the spine in the neutral position and contract the abdominals throughout this sequence.

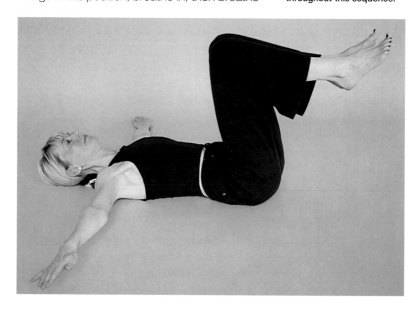

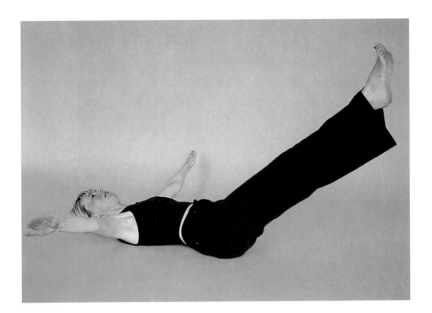

▲ For increased intensity, extend the legs out at a 45-degree angle.

out and start circling the arms, taking them up towards the head, around and out, then down and finally back up to the starting position. Breathe out as you take the arms up and away from the body, inhale as you bring them down and back in. Repeat five times using a smooth, even motion. Keep the arms and shoulders as relaxed as possible, elbows soft, with the shoulderblades drawn down into your back.

3. Breathe in, then breathe out and switch the direction of the arm circles, exhaling as you take the hands down towards the body and out, then inhaling as you bring them up and round. Repeat five times. Change direction again; repeat the sequence one more time, circling five times in one direction and then five in the other. To finish, inhale and lower the arms first, then float the legs back down to the floor, one at a time.

Option

When you are familiar with the above sequence and have developed sufficient strength in the abdominal core, try extending the legs out at a 45-degree angle to the floor as you circle the arms. Lower the legs towards the floor if you want to work the abdominals harder, but make sure that you are able to keep the spine in neutral and the hips stable as you do so. Raise the legs up towards the ceiling for a slightly easier option.

▶ Hamstring stretch

This stretch can be done with your hands grasping the thigh of the extended leg or, for more intensity, with a stretchy exercise band (or small towel) held over the foot.

1. Lie on your back with your spine in neutral, legs bent, knees hip-width apart and your feet parallel. Breathe in and lengthen along the back and neck. Breathe out as you contract the abdominals and lift the right leg to a 90-degree angle, with toes pointed.

2. Breathe in; place your hands around the right thigh. Breathe out and slowly pull the extended leg in towards you. Breathe in and release. Repeat five to ten times, breathing out as you draw the leg in, breathing in as you release. Repeat for the other leg.

> **WATCH OUT!**
>
> Keep your neck relaxed and do not arch the back as you stretch – keep the spine in neutral and contract the abdominals to support the lower back.

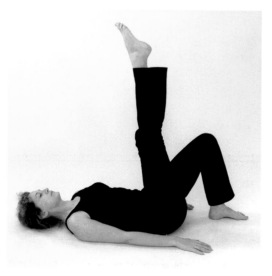

◀ The hamstring stretch can be intensified by extending the leg, with or without the use of an exercise band or hand towel around the foot.

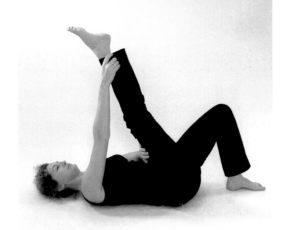

▶ With the leg extended, breathe in and grasp the ankle – or as near to the foot as you can. Exhale and slowly pull the leg in towards you.

Option

1. Follow steps 1 and 2 above, first bringing the knee into the chest to place the exercise band (or hand towel) over the foot and then extending the leg out, flexing the foot.

2. Hold one end of the exercise band in each hand, resting your upper arms and elbows on the floor. Breathe out, contract the abdominal muscles and pull down on the band to add to the intensity of the hamstring stretch.

3. Breathe in and slowly release. Keep the shoulders down and the shoulderblades drawn down into your back. Repeat the hamstring stretch five to ten times, breathing out gradually as you stretch, breathing in as you release. Repeat the sequence for the other leg.

MUST KNOW

Benefits
- Stretches and strengthens the hamstrings.
- Gently stretches the gluteals and the lower back.
- Releases tension in the legs and lower back.

▶ One leg circles

This is designed to improve flexibility in the legs and hips, strengthen the pelvic and abdominal muscles, as well as stretching and developing muscle control.

1. Lie on your back, with your spine in the neutral position, your knees bent and your feet flat on the floor in front of you, approximately hip-width apart.

2. Breathe in, contract your abdominals and breathe out as you lift your left leg in to your chest, until the shin is parallel to the floor, with the knee at a right angle. Place the fingertips of your left hand on your raised knee. Breathe in.

3. Breathe out and, using your fingertips to guide you, circle your knee five to ten times in one direction, and then five to ten times in the other, pausing for a breath, and then breathing out again as you change direction. Keep the opposite leg still, with the knee pointing straight

▼ Rest your fingertips on your raised knee to guide you as you slowly circle the knee. Make sure that the lowered knee remains stable as you work.

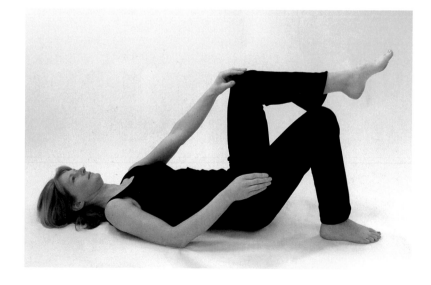

up towards the ceiling. Breathe in, then breathe out as you release the right leg back down to the floor. Repeat for the right leg.

Options

1. Once you can make controlled, smooth circles with your knee, you no longer need your hand to guide you – rest it at your side. Gradually increase the size of the circles, maintaining a slow, even motion in time with the breathing.

2. To increase the difficulty, straighten the raised leg up towards the ceiling and draw the circles with your feet. Keep lengthening the leg out of the hip, away from the body. Keep the knee soft. Circle the leg ten times in one direction, then in the other.

MUST KNOW

Benefits
- Strengthens the pelvic and abdominal muscles.
- Stretches and strengthens the legs.
- Improves flexibility in the legs and hips.

▼ Imagine the circles as coming from the hip joint, rather than the knees, encouraging the hip joint to release as you keep circling.

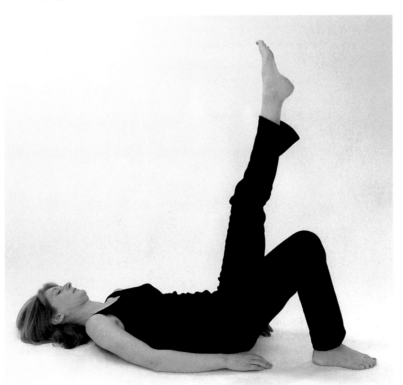

LYING DOWN

▶ Shoulder lifts

When practising this move, keep the shoulders dropped throughout and the neck and shoulders relaxed. Do not tighten your jaw or clench your teeth.

1. Lie on the floor with your back in the neutral position, your legs bent, knees hip-width apart and pointing up to the ceiling, feet in parallel. Rest your arms down by your sides with palms facing downwards. Breathe in as you relax and let the weight of your body sink into the floor as you lengthen along the spine and back of the neck.

2. Breathe out, contract the abdominals a little, keeping the back in neutral, and allow your arms to float up to the ceiling, in line with the shoulders. Keep the arms straight, the elbows soft and the fingers extended.

3. Breathe in and stretch one hand up towards the ceiling, allowing the shoulderblade to lift up and away from the floor very slightly. Breathe out as you drop the shoulderblade back down to the floor, keeping the movement slow and controlled. Repeat, this time stretching the other hand up towards the ceiling.

MUST KNOW

Benefits
• Releases tension in neck, shoulders and upper back.
• Gently mobilizes the shoulder joints and stretches the arms.
• Improves posture and reduces stress.

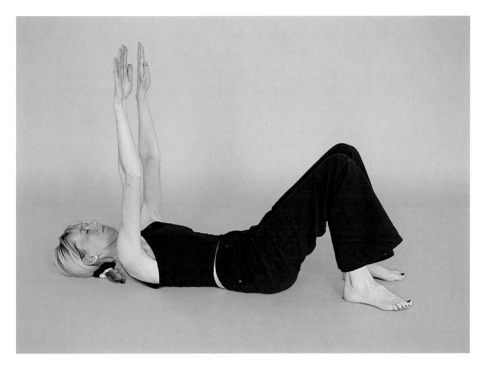

▲ Continue to pull the shoulderblades down into the back, even as you lift the shoulders up away from the floor.

WATCH OUT!

Caution

Take care that you don't tense your neck as you reach upwards with the arms.

4. Repeat the stretch ten times (five times on each side), using alternate arms.

5. Breath in as you lower the arms back down to your sides, keeping the shoulderblades pulled down into the back and the shoulders dropped. Make sure that your face is relaxed throughout the exercise and that you are not clenching your teeth.

▶ Arm openings

As well as having a cushion under your neck, you can also put a small cushion between your knees to help keep your pelvis stable and your knees in alignment in this exercise.

1. Lie on your left side with your knees bent up at right angles to your body, keeping your knees and ankles together. Your back should be in the neutral position, with the spine parallel to the floor – make sure that your waist is lifted slightly, and not dropped to the floor. Place a small cushion under your head to keep your neck in alignment. Position the arms straight out to the side, at just below shoulder level, and place one hand on top of the other.

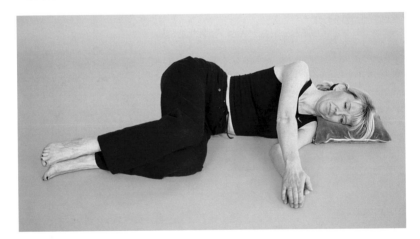

MUST KNOW

Benefits
- Mobilizes and stretches the spine.
- Reduces stiffness and tightness in the back.
- Opens the chest area, gently stretching the arms and neck, and relieving tension.

▲ Place a small cushion under your head to keep your neck in alignment.

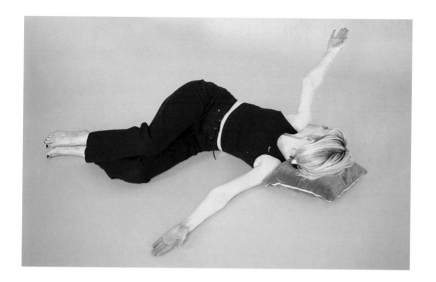

▲ Move the upper body while keeping the lower body still. Only take the arm back as far as you can while maintaining the stability of the hips and legs.

2. Breathe in and lengthen the spine and neck, allowing your weight to sink into the floor, but all the time keeping your back in the neutral position.

3. Breathe out, contract the abdominals and slowly raise the right hand up towards the ceiling then back behind you as far as possible, in a semicircular arc. Keep the arm straight and the elbow soft as you move. Follow the movement of the hand with the eyes, rotating the head and gently stretching the muscles of the neck.

WATCH OUT!

Do not attempt this exercise if you suffer from any back or neck problems or have sustained an injury to the back or neck. If in doubt, consult a doctor.

4. Breathe in as you slowly bring the arm back to the starting position, making sure you keep the abdominals contracted and again following the movement of the hand with the eyes. Keep lengthening through the neck as you move.

5. Repeat five times on this side, then switch positions and repeat the sequence five times lying on the right side.

LYING DOWN

▶ Windmill

**When performing windmills, concentrate on maintaining
the spine in the neutral position and keeping the abdominals
contracted as you move the arms.**

1. Lie on your back with your legs bent, ankles
   hip-width apart, feet flat on the floor. Place
   your arms by your sides. Drop the shoulders,
   drawing the shoulderblades down into your
   back. Check that the spine is in neutral.
   Breathe in, contracting the abdominals, and
   float the arms up to shoulder level, with the
   hands shoulder-width apart, pointing straight
   up to the ceiling, palms facing away from you,
   fingers extended.

2. Breathe out, taking the right arm up behind
   your head, palm up, and the left arm down to
   your side, palm down.

3. In a continuous, even movement, circle the
   right arm out to the side, in the direction
   towards your feet and then back up to the
   starting position, at the same time as you
   circle the left arm out to the side and round

▼ As you breathe out, take
your right arm up behind
the head and your left arm
down to your side.

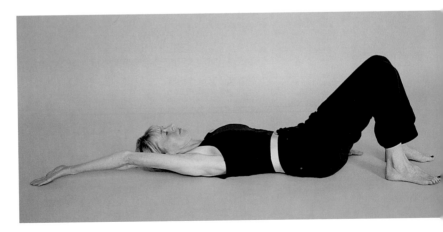

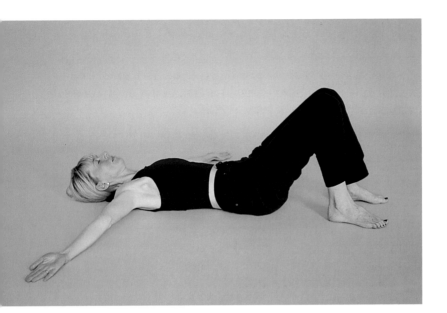

▲ Circle the right arm out to the side, then down towards your feet, at the same time as you circle your left arm out to the side and up towards your head.

MUST KNOW

Benefits
- Mobilizes the muscles of the shoulder area.
- Gently stretches and strengthens the arms.
- Improves co-ordination.

towards your head, then up towards the ceiling, back to the starting position. Keep circling the arms in this sequence for five to ten rotations, breathing out as you take the arms down towards the floor and out to the sides, then breathing in as you bring the arms back to centre.

4. Change the direction of the arms and repeat the sequence.

5. Once you have mastered this exercise, practise changing the direction after each completed rotation.

▶ The Corkscrew

This strength-building exercise demands that you control your movement at every stage of the sequence, even as you move your legs off balance.

1. Lie on your back with your legs stretched straight out in front of you, toes pointing away, knees and ankles together. Rest your arms by your sides, palms to the floor. Check that your spine is in neutral and breathe in.

2. Breathe out as you contract the abdominals and tilt the pelvis forward slightly, tucking the tailbone in. Continue to breathe as you raise your legs up towards the ceiling, keeping the spine in neutral.

3. Using the abdominal contraction to control the lift, squeeze the inner thighs together as you

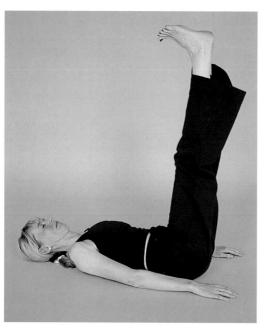

◀ Raise your legs up towards the ceiling, keeping the spine in neutral.

WATCH OUT!

This requires a strong abdominal core and good muscle control, and should only be attempted once you have developed sufficient strength to keep control, even when the move requires you to twist off-centre.

raise your legs, bringing them up and over your head, and slowly peeling the spine away from the floor, one vertebra at a time.

4. Take your legs over behind your head, as far down to the floor as you can, and continue curling up the spine until your weight is resting your shoulders. Press down with your hands to stabilize yourself, if necessary. Keep the legs straight and the knees soft.

5. Keeping legs and hips parallel, breathe in, then breathe out, increase the contraction in the abdominals and slowly draw a circle in the air with the feet, moving them around to the right, then around and down, across, and around and up to the left. Breathe in, breathe out and draw a circle in the opposite direction. Repeat this 'corkscrew' movement five to ten times. To finish, breathe in as you bring the legs back to centre, and out as you lower them to the floor.

MUST KNOW

Benefits
• Improves balance.
• Builds strength.
• Develops muscle control.

▼ Take your legs over behind your head, as far down to the floor as you can manage.

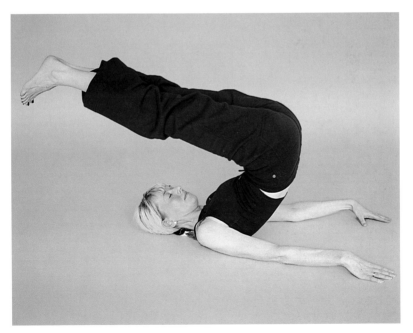

▶ Jack knife

Abdominal strength and flexibility is vital for performing this move, so make sure you have developed sufficient muscle control before attempting this exercise.

1. Lie on your back with your legs extended, feet pointed, knees and ankles together. Let your arms rest by your sides, palms facing downwards. Pull the shoulderblades down and back, making sure the spine is in neutral with the back of the neck lengthened. Focus the eyes straight up at the ceiling.

2. Breathe in, then breathe out as you contract the abdominals and tilt the pelvis forwards. Continuing to breathe out, squeeze the buttocks tightly, squeeze the inner thighs together and lift your feet up towards the ceiling, keeping your legs straight, and your knees soft and toes pointed.

3. Still using the out breath, continue the movement, lowering your feet a few inches (5–8cm) behind your head, taking them straight down towards the floor. Allow your tailbone and lower spine to peel away from the floor, vertebra by vertebra. If necessary, press down with your hands and use your arms to help you balance.

▶ As you breathe out, squeeze the buttocks and inner thighs and lift your feet up towards the ceiling.

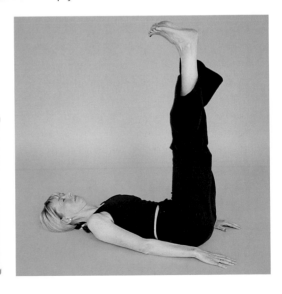

MUST KNOW

Benefits
• Builds strength.
• Improves muscle control.
• Stretches the back, shoulder and arm muscles.

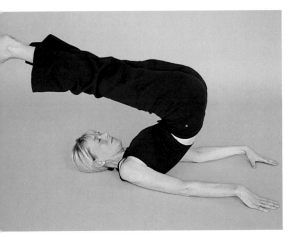

◀ To maximize the strength-building effect, roll down through the spine as slowly as possible, controlling the movement throughout using the abdominal muscles.

WATCH OUT!

- Before you attempt this exercise make sure you have developed sufficient strength in the abdominals and flexibility in the spine. To strengthen your abdominals and muscle control, practise the Rolling up exercise described on pages 94–5.
- Do not attempt this exercise if you have any history of neck or back problems. If you are in any doubt, seek medical advice.
- As you roll up, keep the weight of the body on the shoulders and avoid rolling up onto the neck.

4. When you have gone as far as you can while controlling the move with the abdominal core, breathe in and slowly roll back down through the spine and then lower the legs. Make sure you maintain the abdominal contraction as you roll back down, keeping the move as slow and controlled as possible. Repeat five to ten times.

Option

Once you have mastered the move, you can challenge yourself a little further.

1. Follow the above instructions, this time continuing to peel the spine up away from the floor on the out breath, until your body and legs are in a line pointing straight up towards the ceiling with your weight resting on your shoulders, neck and arms. Control the entire movement with the abdominal core, but, if you need to, use your arms to stabilize yourself.

2. Breathe in and roll back down through the spine to the starting position, keeping the movement slow and controlled. Try to keep your feet positioned directly above your face for as long as possible as you roll down through the spine. Repeat five to ten times.

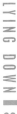

LYING DOWN

▶ Teaser

The aim of this strength-building exercise is to work the upper body without using the legs and arms to help you. Control the movement as you slowly raise and lower the body.

1. Lie on your back with your legs bent, knees hip-width apart and pointing to the ceiling, feet parallel. Place arms by your sides, palms down. Lengthen along the spine and back of the neck.

2. Breathe out, contract the abdominals, and float the hands up towards the ceiling until the arms are parallel to the thighs. At the same time, drop the chin slightly towards the chest and start to roll slowly up through the spine, one vertebra at a time, as far as you can, controlling the move with the abdominals. Keep the shoulders relaxed and the shoulderblades pulled down into your back.

3. Breathe in, contract the abdominals and roll slowly back down through the spine to the floor. Repeat five to ten times.

MUST KNOW

Benefits
- Builds strength in the abdominal core.
- Improves muscle control and stability.
- Increases strength and flexibility in the spine.

▼ Make sure the legs remain still and in position as you roll up and down through the spine.

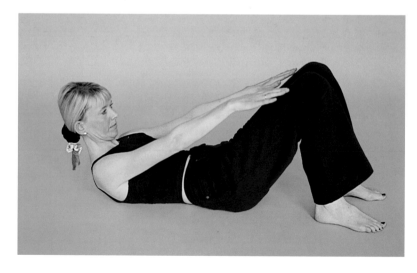

Option 1

Once you are comfortable with the movement, try the sequence keeping one foot on the ground, knee bent, as above, and extending the other leg upwards, squeezing the inner thighs together as you roll up through the spine. Repeat five to ten times, alternating the legs.

Option 2

Repeat the sequence given above, but this time, extend both legs. Keep squeezing the inner thighs together and lengthening the legs away from you as you roll through the spine. If you start to feel your back arching, then raise the legs up towards the ceiling a little, until you feel comfortable once more.

WATCH OUT!

If you feel any pain or discomfort in your lower back, stop immediately and seek medical advice.

▼ When you lengthen both legs away from you, keep squeezing the inner thighs together at all times.

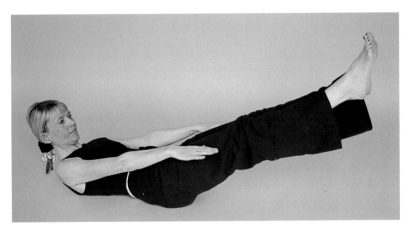

Option 3

Once you have mastered the above technique, try beginning the exercise from a sitting position, extending both legs then lightly grasping the backs of the knees as you slowly roll down through the spine, vertebra by vertebra, as far as you can, keeping the alignment and using the abdominal muscles to control the movement. Breathe in as you roll back up to sitting. Repeat five to ten times, keeping legs raised throughout.

▶ Scissors

As well as building strength in the abdominal core, the back and the legs, this exercise can also improve your concentration and help control your breathing.

1. Lie on the floor with knees bent, hip-width apart, feet parallel, and arms by your sides. Breathe in, checking that your spine is in neutral and your neck and shoulders relaxed.

2. Breathe out, contract the abdominals and float your legs up, one at a time, knees bent, until the thighs are at right angles to the body and shins parallel to the floor.

WATCH OUT!

If you feel any type of pain or discomfort in your lower back or neck, stop immediately and seek medical advice.

▼ Focus on contracting the abdominals, keeping the spine in neutral and the hips level as you 'scissor'.

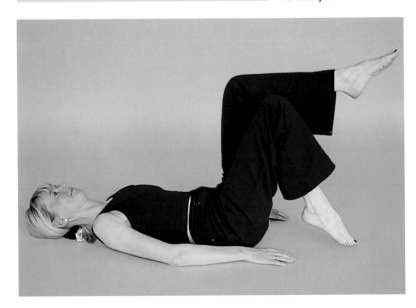

Benefits
- Builds strength in the abdominal core, back and legs.
- Improves concentration and breath control.
- Increases flexibility.

3. Breathe in, keeping your legs in this position, then breathe out and, still keeping the knees bent, 'dip' the toes of one foot down towards the floor, as if into a pool of water, breathe in as you bring the leg back to centre. Repeat five to ten times using alternate legs. You do not need to take the foot all the way to the floor at first – just take it as far as you can while keeping your spine in neutral, your hips level and your abdominals contracted. As you progress you will gradually be able to take the movement further.

Option

1. As your abdominal strength and muscle control develop, gradually extend the legs, increasing the angle of the knee bend little by little, until you are able to do the exercise with completely straight legs, taking one down towards the floor as the other one lifts up. As you move the legs, think of lengthening them away from you, out of the hip joint.

2. At the same time, tuck your chin in to your chest slightly and lengthen along the back of the neck, bringing your head and shoulders up away from the floor. Raise and lower the legs at a controlled, even pace in time with the breathing, changing the breath as you change the direction of the legs. Repeat five to ten times on each leg.

▶ Rolling up

Don't worry if you cannot roll up very far to begin with. The most important element is for you to work the abdominals, keeping the body in the correct alignment. Over time your range of movement will automatically increase.

1. Lie on your back with knees bent, feet flat on the floor hip-width apart. Put your arms by your sides. Drop the shoulders, drawing the shoulderblades down into your back. Check that your spine is in neutral.

2. Breathe in, contract the abdominals, tuck the chin into the chest slightly, lengthen along the back of the neck and allow the head to curl up from the floor. Raise your arms an inch (2–3cm) off the floor, lengthening them away from you, fingers extended, as you begin to roll up. Concentrate on keeping the movement slow, flowing and even. Make sure the shoulders are dropped and keep the shoulderblades pulled down into your back as you roll up through the spine, vertebra by vertebra.

3. When you start to feel resistance in the abdominals and can roll up no further, pause, breathe in, contract the abdominals, then breathe out as you slowly roll back down to the floor, controlling the movement with the abdominals. Repeat five to ten times.

MUST KNOW

Benefits
• Strengthens the abdominals.
• Mobilizes and strengthens the back.
• Improves muscle control.

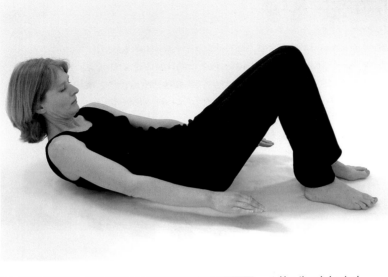

WATCH OUT!

Avoid this exercise if you suffer from any
neck problems.

▲ Use the abdominal
contraction to control
the movement.

Option

1. As an alternative form of rolling up, and to
   increase the intensity of the move, begin
   from the sitting position, with your knees bent
   and your feet flat on the floor in a parallel
   position. Grasp your thighs with your hands,
   arms relaxed.

2. Breathe in, contract the abdominals, tilt
   your pelvis forward slightly and slowly begin
   to curl back, rolling down through the spine.
   When you feel the point of resistance in the
   abdominals, breathe in and return to an
   upright position.

3. Repeat five to ten times, keeping your eyes
   focussed straight in front of you as you curl.

▶ Leg lifts

These exercises can be performed as a sequence: complete the lifts, circles and pulses for one leg before changing position and repeating on the other side.

Single leg lifts

1. Lie on your left side with your left arm extended away from you and your head resting on your arm. Place a small cushion under your head to keep your neck in line with your spine. Bend your knees up to form a right angle with your body and place your right hand, palm down, on the floor by your chest to help you balance. Focus straight in front of you. Breathe in.

MUST KNOW

Benefits

- Strengthens and lengthens the leg muscles.
- Tones and strengthens the buttocks, hips and thighs.
- Mobilizes the hip joint.
- Develops the abdominal core.
- Improves muscle control.

---

2. Breathe out, contract the abdominals and extend the right leg from you, out of the hip joint. Keep the foot flexed as you lengthen down the back of the leg and through the heel. Allow the leg to lift as you lengthen, but keep the extended leg low – raise it an inch or so (2–5cm) from the ground. Do not arch your back or let your waist drop to the floor.

WATCH OUT!

- Do not arch your back as you work – concentrate on keeping the spine in neutral and the back long.
- Keep contracting the abdominals to support your lower back.

Tips

- As your legs grow stronger, you may add light leg weights to increase the intensity of the stretches.
- Keep your back aligned and your spine parallel to the floor – do not allow the waist to drop to the floor as you work the legs.
- Relax the head and neck, allowing the arm (and cushion) to support it.
- Lengthen the lower arm away from you as you work.

3. Breathe in and lower the leg, keeping it straight and in line with the body.

4. Breathe out and extend the leg once more. Repeat five to ten times. To finish, breathe in, breathe out, contract the abdominals and lower the right leg, bending it back up to rest on top of the left leg.

5. Change position and repeat the sequence for the left leg.

▼ The extended leg should only be slightly away from the floor when it is raised.

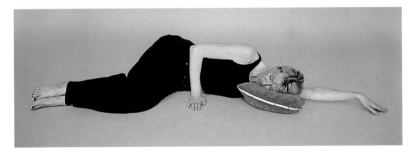

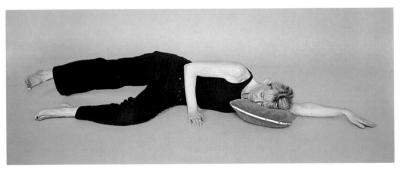

Leg circles

1. Follow the instructions for step 1, page 96.

2. Breathe out, contract the abdominals and extend the right leg away from you, so that it is in line with your hips, parallel to the floor.

3. Holding this position and keeping your breathing slow and even, make small, controlled circles (roughly the size of a coconut) with your leg. Circle five to ten times in one direction and then five to ten times in the other, lengthening the leg away from you, out of the hip joint, as you circle. Again, flex the foot as you lengthen down the back of the leg and out through the heel.

4. Breathe in, then breathe out and lower the right leg, bending the knee and bringing it back to rest on the left leg.

5. Change your position and repeat for the left leg.

▼ Circling movements should be small and controlled.

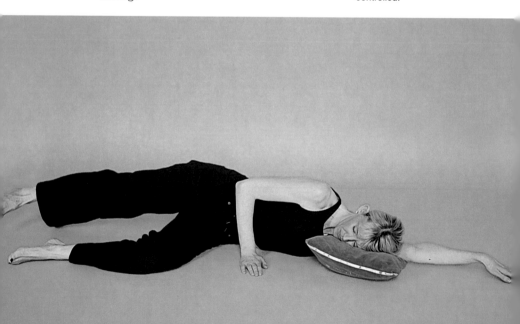

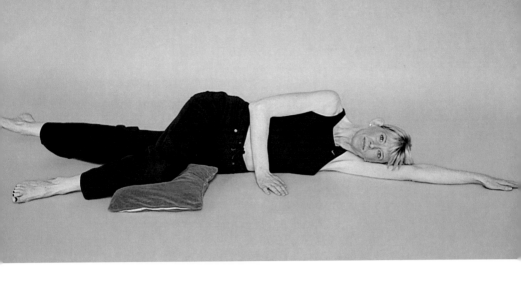

Leg pulses

1. Follow the instructions as steps 1 and 2 of the leg circles exercise on page 98.

2. Breathe out and 'pulse' the extended leg down an inch or two (2–5cm) and then back up again – do not raise it higher than the level of your hips.

3. Pulse the leg 10 to 20 times in total, changing the breathing every five counts.

4. Breathe in, then breathe out as you lower the leg back to the starting position.

5. Change position and repeat for the left leg.

Option – lower leg pulses

1. Still lying on your left side with your left arm extended away from you, your head resting on your left arm and your right hand on the floor in front of you to help you balance and your knees bent up at right angles, place a cushion under your right knee to raise it slightly off the ground and prevent you from tilting your hip forwards.

▲ Another option for leg pulses involves extending your lower leg out along the ground at an angle of 45 degrees to the body.

2. Extend your left leg out along the ground at an angle of 45 degrees to the body. Focus your eyes straight out in front of you. Breathe in.

3. Breathe out, contract your abdominals and pulse the left leg up away from the ground a total of 10 to 20 times, changing the breath every five counts as before.

4. Breathe in and bend your left leg back to join your right leg.

5. Change your position and repeat for the right leg.

Option – arm position

Once you have developed sufficient stability, muscle control and strength in the abdominal core, try resting your uppermost arm along the side of the body as you perform these leg exercises. If you start to wobble, however, or lose your balance, place your hand back

▼ Challenge yourself with the uppermost arm resting along the side of the body, and extend the bottom leg along the floor.

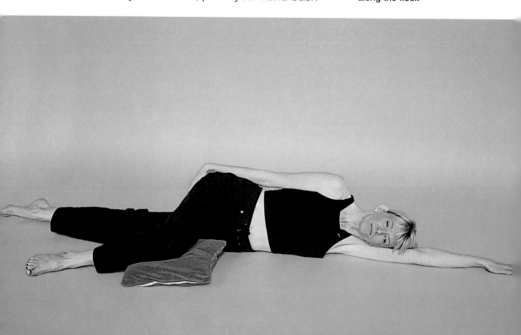

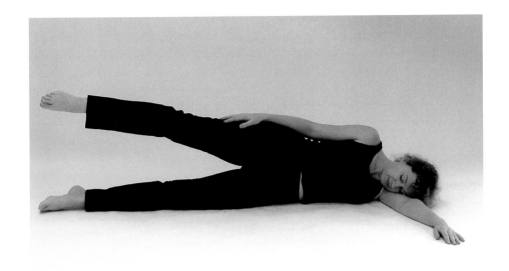

down on the floor in front of you. This shows that you are not yet ready for this particular variation and need to continue practising the basic exercise.

Option – leg position

When you have mastered the leg-lift sequence, keeping the bottom leg bent up at a right angle, try making this sequence of exercises a little more challenging for you by extending the bottom leg along the floor, in line with the body. You will need to work harder to keep control and stability in this position. If you find you are struggling and unable to maintain the correct alignment, return to the previous version.

▲ Once you have gained sufficient strength and control, try extending the supporting leg. Keep contracting the abdominals and maintain your spine in neutral as you work.

▶ Double leg lifts (side)

Once you have mastered the single leg lifts, practising double leg lifts will intensify the effect on the abdominals, hips, buttocks and leg muscles.

1. Lie on your left side with your body in a straight line, knees and ankles together. Rest your left arm along the floor, to support the head. (Alternatively, place a small cushion under your head to support it, if you prefer.) Position the right arm along the side of your body or, if you need to, place your right hand on the floor in front of you to help maintain your balance.

2. Check that your spine is in the neutral position with your shoulders and hips aligned. Lift your waist up away from the floor to keep the spine in its correct alignment. Breathe in.

3. Breathe out, contract the abdominals and, keeping your knees and ankles together, squeeze the inner thighs together and

▼ Avoid tilting the shoulder or hip forward as you extend and raise the legs.

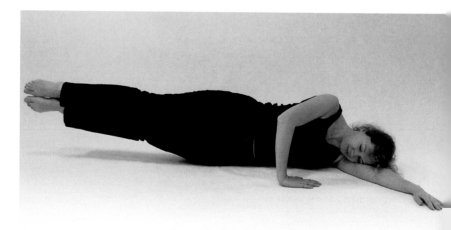

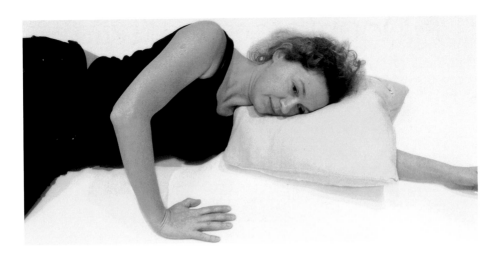

slowly extend both legs, allowing them to raise up away from the floor. Make sure that your legs remain in line with your body. The toes should be softly pointed. Concentrate on keeping your back in the neutral position as you raise the legs away from the floor.

▲ If your neck feels uncomfortable, place a small cushion under your head for support.

4. Breathe in and lower the legs, but do not bring them all the way back down to the floor. Repeat five to ten times. Change position and repeat for the other side.

Option

To increase the intensity of the movement, breathe out as you raise the legs, then hold this position and breathe in, then breathe out as you lower the legs.

MUST KNOW

Benefits
• Works the abdominals, the hips, the buttocks and the leg muscles.
• Increases strength.
• Improves muscle control.

▶ Inner thigh stretch

If you suffer from stiffness around the hip and pelvic areas, this is a wonderful stretching exercise that will gradually improve your mobility and flexibility in this particular area.

1. Lie on your back with your knees bent. Inhale and lengthen through the spine and neck. Float your legs up, one at a time, keeping your knees bent. Rest your hands on your knees and let the knees gradually drop out to the sides. Inhale and lengthen along the spine and neck, concentrating on dropping your shoulders away from your ears and drawing the shoulderblades down and back behind you.

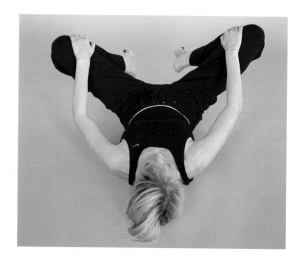

▶ Gently pull the knees apart, increasing the stretch to the inner thighs as you go.

MUST KNOW

Benefits
- Stretches the inner thigh muscles.
- Releases tension in the lower back, hips and pelvic area.
- Rebalances the pelvis.

WATCH OUT!

Do not pull the knees too far out to the sides – let gravity do most of the work for you.

2. Breathe out, contract the abdominals and gently pull the knees apart, gradually increasing the stretch to the inner thighs. Inhale and release. Repeat this stretch five to ten times, increasing the intensity of the stretch little by little each time. Breathe out as you stretch the legs apart and breathe in as you release. Stay centred at all times and avoid rolling to one side of the other as you perform the movement. Keep the tailbone in contact with the floor and allow the weight of the legs to create the initial stretch, releasing through the hips.

▼ For a more intense stretch, straighten the legs and gently pull them apart as you breathe out.

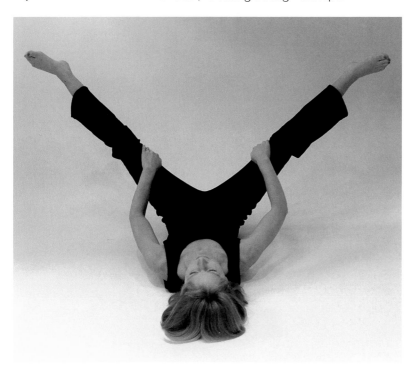

▶ Rolling over

**Practising this exercise will improve flexibility of the spine
and stretch the shoulder and neck areas. However, avoid
this if you suffer from any neck or lower back problems.**

1. Lie on your back with your knees bent, feet
   flat on the floor, hip-width apart, and your
   spine in neutral. Rest your arms by your sides,
   palms facing down.

2. Breathe in, then breathe out, contract the
   abdominals and float the legs up, one at a
   time, keeping the knees at right angles to the
   body, shins parallel to the floor. Breathe in.

3. Breathe out and slowly lower your feet
   straight down towards your face as far as
   possible, straightening your legs, but keeping
   your spine on the floor.

▼ Keeping your spine on
the floor, lower your feet
down towards your face as
far as possible.

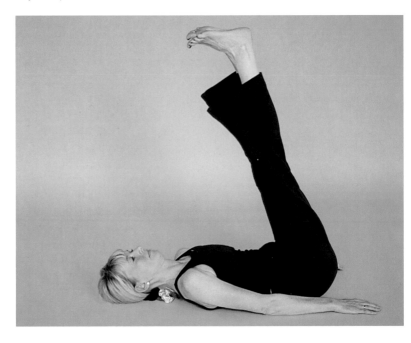

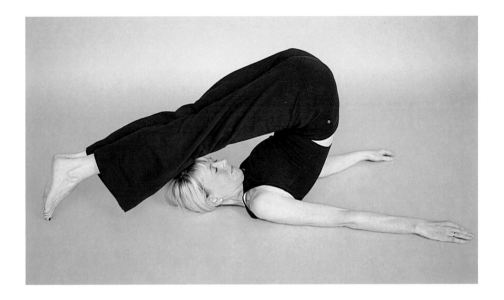

4. Continue the movement as you exhale, taking your feet over your head, allowing the spine to peel away from the floor, one vertebra at a time. If necessary, press down into the floor with your arms to stabilize yourself. Don't worry if you are unable to take your feet all the way to the floor at this stage, just take them as far as you can, trying to increase the stretch a little more each time. When you have reached as far as you can, breathe in.

5. Breathe out, contract the abdominals and roll slowly back down through the spine, vertebra by vertebra. Use the abdominal muscles to control the move as you work against gravity and roll back down. Bend the knees a little if you find it too hard to keep your legs straight for this section of the movement.

6. Once your tailbone is in contact with the floor, bring the legs back so that the feet are pointing straight up to the ceiling. Repeat the sequence five to ten times.

▲ If you are able, take your feet all the way down to the floor.

MUST KNOW

Benefits
- Improves the flexibility of the spine.
- Strengthening the abdominals.
- Increases muscle control.
- Stretches the hamstring, shoulder and neck areas.

▶ Ankle circles

A wonderful exercise to ease tired and aching feet and legs at the end of the day. Your ankles will become more flexible and the circulation in your legs will also improve.

1. Lie on your back with your legs bent, knees pointing up to the ceiling, feet in parallel.

2. Keeping your spine in neutral and your hips level and in line with your shoulders, breathe in, contract the abdominals, then exhale and float the right leg upwards, bending your knee in towards your chest and extending the right foot towards the ceiling. Check that your ankle is in line with your hip and you have not taken the leg out too far or in towards the centre.

3. Grasp your right thigh with both hands, to make sure that the leg remains still as you flex and rotate the feet. Bend your arms and point your elbows out to the sides.

▼ Float the right leg upwards as you exhale, extending the right foot towards the ceiling.

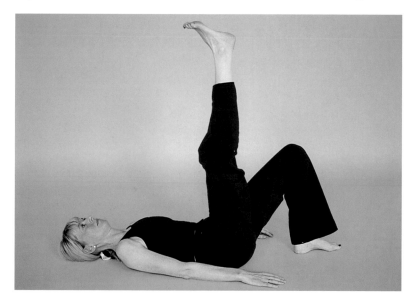

Benefits
- Strengthens and stretches the ankles.
- Relieves tired feet and legs.
- Improves circulation in the legs.

4. Slowly flex your right foot in towards your face then release it back, making the entire movement as smooth as possible. Repeat five to ten times.

5. Now, maintaining this position, circle the foot five to ten times in one direction, then five to ten times in the opposite direction.

6. Breathe out, contract your abdominals and lower your right foot back down on to the floor.

7. Repeat the same sequence of movements for the left leg.

▼ Flex your foot slowly towards your face, then back again, keeping the movement smooth and even.

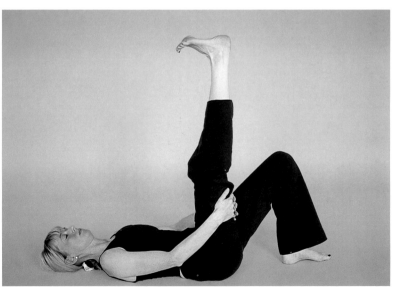

▶ Pillow squeeze 1

This is an excellent exercise to finish with at the end of your routine, as it relieves tension in the lower back and pelvic area. Concentrate as well on relaxing the face and jaw.

1. Lie on your back with your knees bent, feet flat on the floor, knees and ankles together. Place a cushion or pillow between your knees. Rest your hands on your ribs with your elbows pointing out to the side. Breathe in.

▼ With a cushion between your knees, rest your hands on your ribs and breathe in.

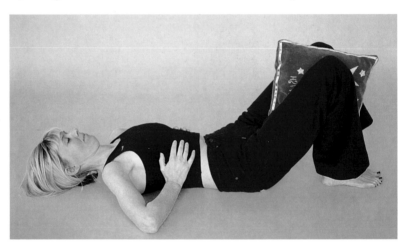

MUST KNOW

Tips
- Maintain the back in neutral as you squeeze, keeping the tailbone in contact with the floor.
- Keep the ribs down as you squeeze – placing your hands on your ribs will allow you to check that you are not lifting them.
- Make sure that your neck and shoulders are relaxed and that you are not clenching your jaw.
- Focus on squeezing the knees together – do not tighten the buttocks or the hip area.
- Once you are confident that you can squeeze without lifting the ribs, then position the arms at your sides, palms down.

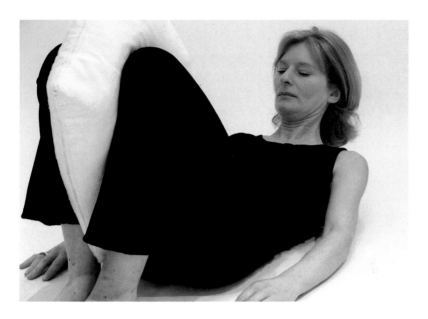

▲ Once confident, position the arms at your sides, palms down, and slowly raise your head off the floor as you squeeze.

MUST KNOW

Benefits
- Strengthens the inner thighs.
- Improves pelvic alignment.
- Releases tension in the lower back and buttocks.

2. Breathe out, contract the abdominals and squeeze the cushion with your knees. Hold for a count of ten, continuing to breathe out as you squeeze. Breathe in and release. Repeat five times.

3. As you are performing this exercise, continue to focus on your breathing and allow your body to relax. When first carrying out this exercise, most of us have a tendency to clench the jaw or tighten the buttocks. Concentrate on remaining relax and soft, while focussing on contracting the abdominal core.

want to know more?

Take it to the next level...

Go to...
▶ **The neutral position** – page 31
▶ **Abdominals** – pages 168–9

Have a go...
▶ **Think 'activity' instead of 'exercise'** any movement is good for you, even more so if you enjoy it, too – plan some fun activities with friends and family
▶ **Autogenic training** is a highly effective relaxation technique. Try http://www.hscti.com/autogenic/

Other sources
▶ **Meditation websites and CD-Roms** for sample meditations and information

facing

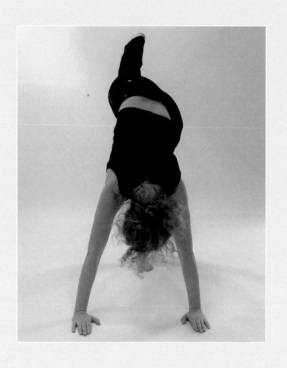

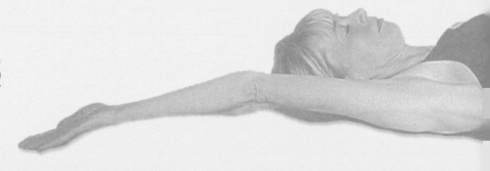

down

As in the previous chapter, the body is supported by the floor. All the exercises in this group are designed to build strength and flexibility in the abdominals and the upper and lower back, as well as developing greater flexibility throughout the entire spine.

Horizontal star

When performing this move you should feel comfortable, so place a small cushion or towel under your forehead if necessary, and contract the abdominals as you stretch.

1. Lie face down on the floor. Legs and arms should be slightly wider than hip- or shoulder-width apart so you lie on the floor in a 'star' position.

2. Drop your shoulders down away from your ears and pull your shoulderblades down into your back.

3. Breathe in and lengthen along the spine and neck.

4. Breathe out, contract the abdominals and lengthen the right arm and the left leg, raising them off the ground very slightly and keeping the elbows soft as you stretch.

5. Breathe in and release back down. Repeat for the other arm and leg.

6. Repeat the sequence five to ten times, using opposite arms and legs each time, and alternating with each repetition.

▼ Keep lengthening the neck as you extend the arms and legs.

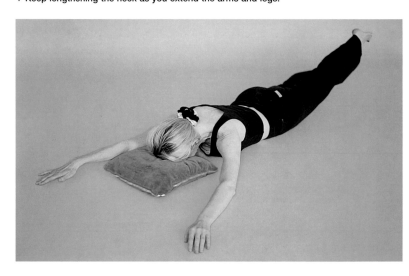

FACING DOWN

Dart

Work both sides of the body evenly with this exercise, keeping your shoulders and hips parallel as you lift. Try to avoid leaning to one side as you raise up.

1. Lie on your front with your legs straight, big toes together, heels dropped out to the sides. Rest your head on the floor, facing to one side. Place your arms by your sides, fingers extended downwards. Breathe in and lengthen along the spine and the back of the neck.

2. Breathe out, contract the abdominals, drop the shoulders and pull the shoulderblades into your back as you raise the upper body using the muscles of the upper back. Keep the neck long; focus your eyes forward and down. As you lift the upper body, allow the hands to lift up slightly and reach the fingertips towards your feet, palms facing in towards the body. At the same time bring the heels in and squeeze the inner thighs together.

3. Keeping your abdominals contracted, your shoulders dropped and your shoulderblades pulled down, breathe in and relax back down, allowing your heels to drop back out to the sides and resting your forehead on the floor, but this time facing to the other side. Repeat five times.

Option

To increase the intensity, breathe out as you raise up, hold the position as you breathe in, then breathe out, contracting the abdominals as you go down.

▼ As you lift the upper body, reach the fingertips, palms facing inwards, towards the feet.

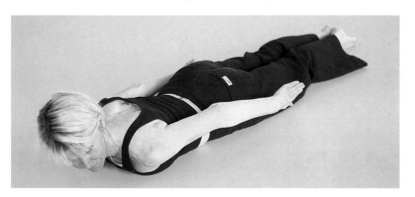

Shoulder press

This exercise works the upper back and shoulders without involving the muscles of the lower body. Allow the legs and buttocks to stay soft as you raise and lower the upper body.

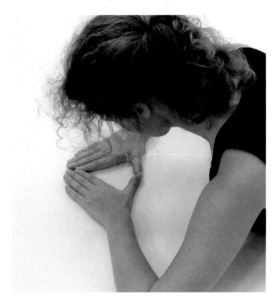

◄ Place your hands in a triangle shape, or one on top of the other, just slightly in front of your head.

1. Lie on your front with your legs straight, knees and ankles slightly apart, forehead resting on the floor, your hands placed, either one on top of each other or forming a triangle, slightly above your head, elbows pointing out to the sides. Lengthen along the spine and the back of the neck. Breathe in.

MUST KNOW

Benefits
- Strengthens the upper back.
- Releases tension in the neck and shoulders.
- Improves posture and alignment.
- Increases muscle control.

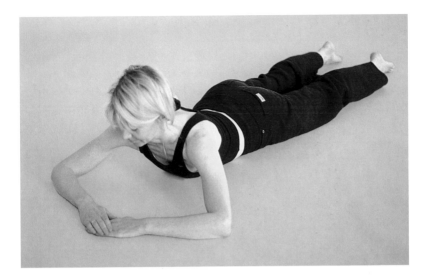

▲ Do not push down on your hands as you raise up. Try lifting them off the floor without changing your body position.

2. Breathe out, contract the abdominals, drop the shoulders and pull the shoulderblades down into your back as you raise the upper body away from the floor, using the muscles of the upper back. Keep your hands in position on the floor, but do not push down on them as you raise up or use them to support you – you should be able to lift them off the floor without changing the position of your body.

3. Keeping your abdominals contracted, your shoulders dropped and your shoulderblades pulled down, breathe in and relax back down, resting your forehead back on the floor. Work both sides of the body evenly, keeping your shoulders and hips parallel to each other as you raise and lower the upper body evenly. Keep your spine and neck lengthened and the abdominals contracted. Repeat five times. If you regularly spend time at a computer, behind a desk or at the wheel of a vehicle, take a few minutes each day to carry out the shoulder press. You will feel the benefits almost immediately.

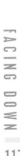

FACING DOWN

117

Heel kicks

This exercise is excellent for stretching the inner thigh muscles. The arms and chest muscles are also strengthened when taking the move further by performing Option 2.

1. Lie face down, with your neck lengthened and forehead resting on your hands, elbows pointing out to the sides, your legs in parallel and slightly apart. Breathe in.

2. Breathe out, contract the abdominals and kick the right heel towards the right buttock, making sure that the hips and thighs remain in contact with the floor. Release the leg slightly then kick once more.

WATCH OUT!

- Do not attempt this exercise if you suffer from any knee or back problems.
- If you suffer from knee stiffness, try stretching the heel slowly towards the buttock, instead of kicking.

▼ Keep lengthening along the spine and back of the neck as you kick the heels.

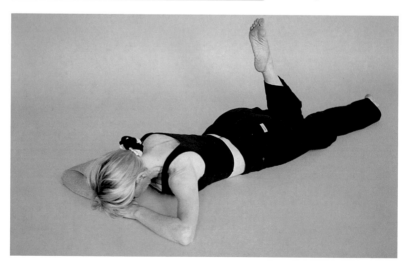

MUST KNOW

Benefits
- Stretches the thigh muscles.
- Strengthens arms, chest muscles, hip flexors and hamstrings.

3. Breathe in and lower the right leg, lengthening the knee away from the hip as you lower.

4. Repeat for the left leg, then repeat the entire sequence five to ten times.

Option 1

To intensify the stretch, flex the raised foot as you kick the heel towards the buttock.

Option 2

For a more challenging version of this exercise, repeat the move with your head lifted up away from your hands, your shoulders dropped and your upper body supported on your forearms. Lengthen along the spine and back of the neck, and focus your eyes down to your hands.

▼ For greater intensity, perform the sequence with your head lifted away from your hands.

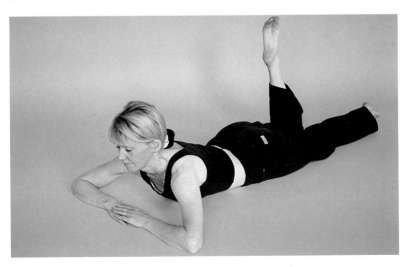

Leg pull

Keep the hips and shoulders level throughout this sequence. Don't let your hips sink towards the floor as you raise the leg and don't raise your bottom higher than your shoulders.

1. Position yourself face down on your hands and knees with your forearms resting on the floor, your hips and shoulders level and your toes tucked under, feet slightly apart. Focus your eyes straight down to the floor, drop your shoulders away from your ears and draw your shoulderblades down into your back. Breathe in and lengthen along the spine and back of the neck.

2. Breathe out, contract your abdominals and extend your left leg straight up behind you, keeping the left knee soft and the foot flexed. Keep your hips level throughout – lengthen the left leg out of the hip joint as you lift, but do not let the left hip raise up too.

▼ Focus your eyes straight down to the floor to help stabilize you.

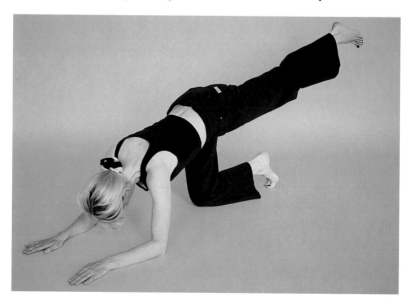

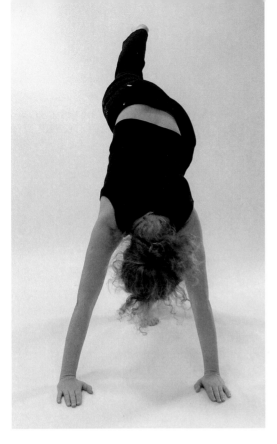

Benefits
- Strengthens the abdominals, the back, the shoulders and the arms.
- Stretches and strengthens the legs.
- Improves balance and stability.

◄ A more challenging version of this exercise is to raise yourself up onto your hands and feet, straightening your arms and legs.

3. Breathe in and lower the left leg, continuing to lengthen down the back of the leg and out through the heel as you do so. Repeat the lift five times with the left leg, then switch legs and repeat five times with the right.

Option

Once you have developed sufficient strength and stability in the abdominals and upper body, you can try this challenging variation. Repeat the exercise, this time straightening your arms and legs and raising yourself up onto your hands and feet. Check that your hands are directly below your shoulders. Keep lengthening along the back of the neck. Breathe out, contract the abdominals and raise the legs in turn, as before.

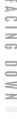

FACING DOWN

121

▶ Plank

As you perform this movement, keep your body stabilized throughout and ensure that the abdominal muscles are contracted. If you feel any pain, stop immediately.

1. Position yourself face down with your forearms resting on the floor, hands either side of your shoulders, feet hip-width apart. Drop your shoulders and draw your shoulderblades down into your back. Lengthen along the spine and neck. Focus your eyes straight down to the floor in front of you and breathe in.

2. Breathe out and contract your lower abdominals as you lift up onto your knees and hands, keeping your eyes focussed downwards and your spine and neck lengthened.

3. Still using the out breath, tuck your toes under and raise yourself up away from the floor, keeping your legs straight, your spine lengthened and your shoulderblades drawn down into your back. As you lift yourself up, do not raise

MUST KNOW

Benefits
- Strengthens the abdominals, the lower back, the upper body, the arms and the legs.
- Opens out the chest and strengthens chest muscles.
- Improves balance and posture.
- Develops core stability.
- Releases tension in the neck and shoulders.

Do not attempt this exercise if you suffer from any problems with your neck, back or wrists. Seek medical advice if you are in any doubt.

your hips any higher than your shoulders or drop them down towards the floor. Do not swing or use the body's momentum to achieve the movement. If you are new to exercise or find this position too challenging, perform the exercise on your knees until you build up more strength. Breathe in as you lower yourself back down to the floor. Repeat this sequence five to ten times. Regularly practising the plank movement will improve your balance and posture, as well as developing core stability and strength throughout your entire body.

▼ Keep your hips level and the spine lengthened as you raise yourself up away from the floor.

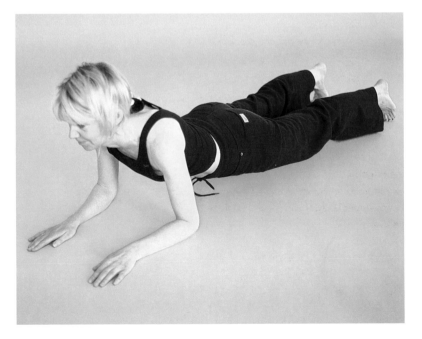

FACING DOWN

Swan position

Keep the neck and spine lengthened throughout this sequence and the abdominals contracted to support the lower back.

1. Lie face down with your forehead resting on the floor, and your legs and arms stretched away from you, slightly wider than hip- or shoulder-width apart. Your feet should be softly pointed and your elbows slightly bent.

2. Drop the shoulders away from your ears and pull the shoulderblades into the back. Breathe in.

MUST KNOW

Benefits
- Strengthens the back and legs.
- Increases strength and flexibility in the upper back, arms and shoulders.
- Tones the buttocks, thighs and hips.
- Improves muscle control.

▼ To begin, lie face down on the floor with your legs and arms stretched away from you.

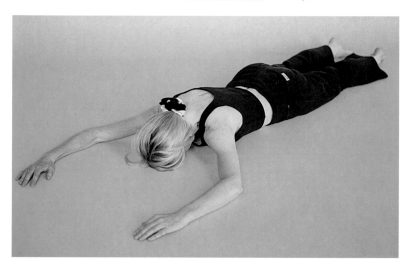

3. Breathe out, contract the abdominals and, keeping your eyes focussed down to the ground, lengthen up through the chest and raise the upper body slightly, keeping the forearms in contact with the floor. Breathe in and lower the body back down. Repeat five times.

4. Breathe out, contract the abdominals, lengthen through the chest, raising the upper body away from the floor and this time allowing the arms to raise up from the floor slightly. Breathe in and lower. Repeat five times.

5. Now, keeping your forehead in contact with the floor, adjust your hand position, so that your hands are palms down, slightly above your shoulders. Breathe out, contract the abdominals, and, without moving the arms or head, lengthen the legs away from you, squeezing the buttocks and allowing the legs to raise up from the floor a little. Breathe as you release the legs back down. Repeat five times.

▼ Keeping the forearms in contact with the floor, lengthen through the chest and raise the upper body.

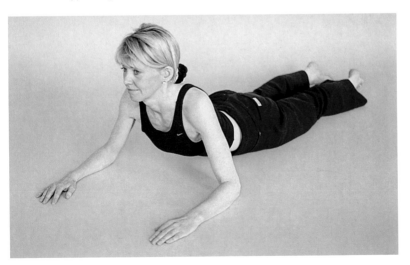

▶ Side bend

The abdominals are essential in this exercise as they provide strength, control and stability to the torso. Regular practice will also develop improved balance.

1. Sit on your right side with your knees bent, legs in parallel, knees, ankles and feet together. Place your right forearm on the floor, elbow directly below the shoulder and the hand pointing straight out. Rest your left arm on the floor in front of you. Keep your eyes focussed forwards throughout this exercise.

2. Breathe in, lengthen spine and neck and lift the ribs slightly.

3. Breathe out, contract the abdominals and raise your hips up away from the floor until the body is in a straight line, with the torso and the

▼ Do not allow your weight to sink into your wrist and shoulder.

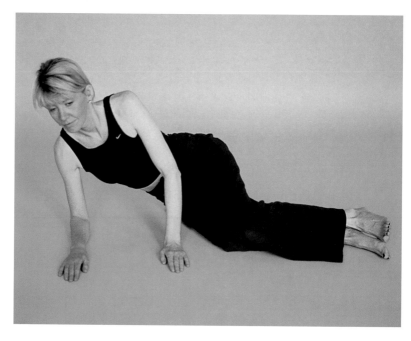

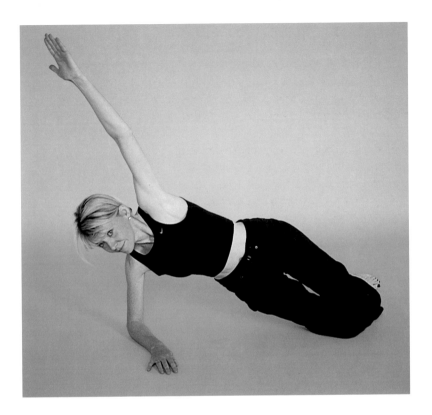

▲ As you stretch, avoid
tilting the uppermost
shoulder forward or
arching the back.

upper right arm forming a triangle with the
floor. If this is too difficult for you to achieve at
this stage, lift the hips as high as you can,
keeping the movement controlled. Use the
fingertips of the left hand to help you balance.
Try to avoid letting the hips drop to the floor or
tilt forward as you lift the torso up away from
the floor.

4. Breathe in, check that your shoulders are
   dropped and draw the shoulderblades down
   into the back. Keeping the pressure on the
   right elbow and knee, breathe out, contract
   the abdominals and allow the left arm to curve
   slowly upwards and over your head, creating
   a stretch along the left side of the body. The
   left elbow should be soft and the hand

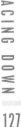

MUST KNOW

Benefits
• Improves muscle control and balance.
• Increases flexibility.
• Stretches the waistline and hips.

relaxed. Only take the arm as far as you can while keeping the movement controlled and the body in alignment.

5. Breathe in as you bring the arm back down and lower the hips to the floor.

6. Repeat five to ten times then change sides and repeat the sequence.

Option 1

If you find it too difficult to maintain your balance and lift the arm at the same time, practise the exercise just lifting and lowering the hips. As your balance improves and you gain confidence, try adding the arm movement once more.

Option 2

Once you have developed sufficient strength and control, try the exercise with the legs extended and the left foot crossed over the right ankle and placed flat down on the floor. Raise yourself up off the ground, pressing down into the floor with your right hand and your left foot, straightening the right arm and making sure that the spine and neck are aligned.

▲ Option 2 should only be attempted once you have developed sufficient strength and control.

WATCH OUT!

Do not attempt this exercise if you suffer from any wrist or shoulder problems.

FACING DOWN

Pillow squeeze 2

Like the first pillow squeezing exercise on page 110, this is an excellent exercise to finish with at the end of a routine. Relax your neck and make sure you do not clench your jaw.

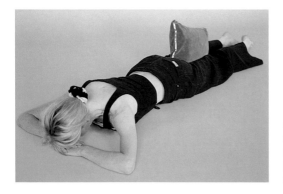

◀ Lengthen out of the hips and down through the legs and feet as you work the buttocks, inner thighs and abdominal core.

1. Lie on your front with a cushion placed between your thighs. Position your feet so that they are pointing away from the body with the toes together and the heels dropped out to the side. Make sure that your back is straight, with your hips and shoulders parallel to each other and not tilting to one side. Check that your hips are level, with both hips in contact with the floor. Place your hands, one on top of the other, palms down, on the floor, under your forehead, elbows pointing out to the sides. Drop your shoulders away from your ears. Breathe in.

2. Breathe out, contract the abdominals (drawing them up away from the floor very slightly, but keeping the back in neutral) and squeeze the cushion together with your inner thighs, tightening the buttocks and pressing your heels in together as you. Hold for a count of five then breathe in and release, allowing the heels to drop out to the sides once more. Repeat the squeeze five times.

want to know **more?**

Take it to the next level...

Go to...
▶ **Horizontal star** – page 172
▶ **Press ups** – page 177

Have a go...
▶ **Eating well**
a nutritious, balanced diet is essential for a healthy body
▶ **Exercise outdoors**
take your mat to the park, or even the beach, for an uplifting Pilates session

Other sources
▶ **Internet sites like www.oprah.com**
see 'mind and body' for a range of fitness information and suggestions

sitting &

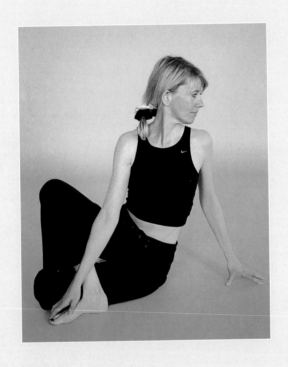

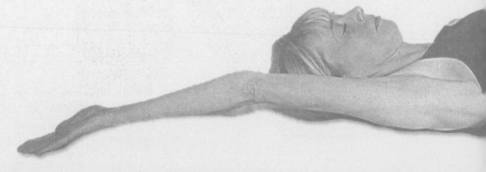

kneeling

When performing mat work in a sitting or kneeling position, remember to keep the abdominals – the body's powerhouse – contracted as you work. This will prevent you from placing undue stress on the muscles of the lower back and unnecessary pressure on the spine.

▶ Spine stretch

This particular exercise works on the spine and enhances good posture. It also stretches your hamstrings and opens out the shoulder area.

MUST KNOW

Benefits
- Mobilizes and stretches the spine.
- Releases tension in the back.
- Stretches the hamstrings.

1. Sit tall, in an upright position on the floor, with your legs slightly apart, open to slightly wider than your hips' width. and your spine and neck lengthened. Relax and focus on releasing any tension held in the back. Straighten your legs, but keep your knees

▼ Keep the legs as straight as possible throughout this movement, but do not lock the knees.

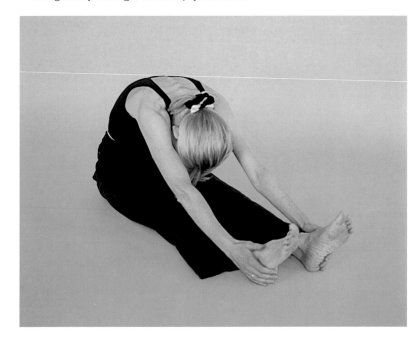

soft. Rest your hands on your thighs. Breathe in and sit up even taller, as if the crown of your head was being pulled by an invisible string up through the ceiling.

2. Breathe out, contract the abdominals, tilt the pelvis forward slightly and lengthen the back up out of the hips.

3. Still using the out breath, drop your chin slightly towards your chest and curve forwards and down towards your thighs, rolling down through the spine one vertebra at a time. Imagine you are forming the letter 'C' with your body. Allow the hands to slide gradually forwards along your legs towards your feet as you slowly stretch out. Keep your shoulders down and your shoulderblades drawn down into your back. Try not to collapse the ribs at the front of the body as you curve the body over – think of lifting your torso over a large inflatable beach ball.

4. Breathe in and reverse the exercise, rolling up as if constrained by a wall behind you. Breathe out as you return to the seated position.

5. Repeat the sequence three to five times.

MUST KNOW

Tips
- Choose whether you do this exercise with flexed or pointed feet. The flexed-foot position will give a more intense stretch in the backs of the legs.
- If your hamstrings are very tight and you find it too uncomfortable to sit with your legs extended, then bend your knees a little (drawing your feet in towards the body), place the soles of your feet together and drop your knees out to the side.

▶ Spine twist

Keep lifting up out of the pelvis and lengthening at the waist as you rotate the spine. The head should remain in line with the body to avoid twisting the neck too far round as you stretch.

1. Sit on the floor with your legs fairly wide apart. Drop your shoulders away from your ears and draw your shoulderblades down into your back. Breathe in, contract your abdominals, tilt your pelvis forward slightly and raise your arms to just below shoulder level, so that they are parallel to your legs. Keep the arms straight and the elbows soft.

2. Exhale and twist your upper body round to the right, so that your torso is parallel to the right leg. Breathe in and release to come back to centre, then breathe out and twist the upper body to the left this time. Breathe in and return to centre once more.

3. Repeat the sequence five to ten times on each side, trying to increase the stretch ever so slightly each time. Regular practice of this spine twisting exercise will gradually improve flexibility in the upper back, as well as relieve any tightness that may be held in the spine. An added benefit with this exercise is that the inner thighs are also gently stretched.

MUST KNOW

Benefits
- Mobilizes and strengthens the upper back.
- Improves flexibility.
- Relieves tightness in the spine.
- Gently stretches the inner thighs.

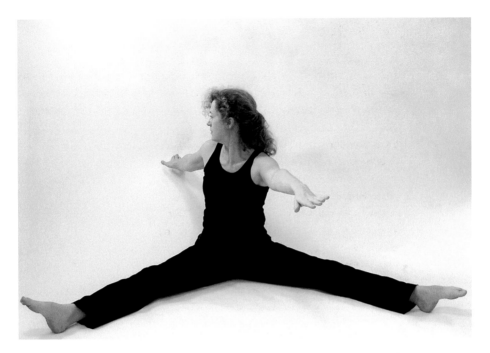

▲ Do not allow the upper body to collapse as you twist round.

WATCH OUT!

Sit with your legs as wide apart as you can, but making sure that the position is comfortable for you – remember, the purpose of this exercise is to work the upper body, not to stretch the inner thighs.

Option

For a slightly more challenging stretch, repeat the above sequence, but this time once you have twisted the torso round to the right, lengthen your left arm forward over your right leg towards the foot, taking your right arm back behind you. Do not collapse the upper body as you stretch forwards – think of stretching over an imaginary beach ball. Your hips should remain stationary and your legs and feet relaxed. Breathe in and return to centre then repeat for the other side.

▶ Rolling back

The most important element in this exercise is to make sure that the abdominals control the rolling back movement – not the momentum of the body.

1. Sit on the floor with your legs bent, knees and ankles together, feet flat on the floor. Keep your shoulders down and relaxed. Sit straight but not stiff or tense. Place your hands, palms down, on the floor, either side of your hips. Breathe in.

2. Breathe out, contract your abdominals, tilt your pelvis forward and slowly start to roll back, keeping your hands on the floor beside you, tucking your chin in to your chest, lengthening your neck and focussing your eyes straight ahead. At all times control the movement so it does not feel jerky.

3. Continue rolling back down to the floor, allowing your feet to come away from the floor and tucking your knees into your chest. Make sure the movement is as smooth and even as you can make it, if possible in time with the breathing.

4. Breathe in and roll back up to a sitting position, still keeping your abdominals

MUST KNOW

Benefits
• Works the abdominals.
• Mobilizes the lower back.
• Improves muscle control.

WATCH OUT!

• If your lower back is tight or stiff, or you find this exercise too difficult, focus on the Rolling up exercise instead (pages 94–5) to improve your strength before trying this.
• Do not attempt this exercise if you have any neck problems or any discomfort in the neck and shoulders.

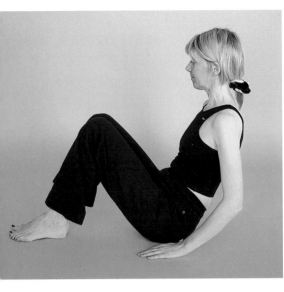

◄ Contract your abdominals and start to slowly roll back, keeping the movement controlled and smooth.

▼ Continue to roll back down to the floor, bringing your knees in towards your chest.

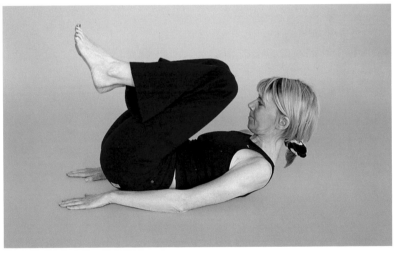

contracted, your knees tucked in towards your chest and allowing the momentum of the movement – in conjunction with the abdominal muscles – to bring you back. Press down with your hands to help you, if necessary, particularly if you do not feel stabilized during the movement. Repeat the exercise five to ten times.

Rolling like a ball

A challenging move and one that will really improve your abdominal control. If you find it too hard, practise Rolling back (pages 136–7) until it seems easy, then go on to this move.

1. Sit on the floor with your legs bent, knees and ankles together, feet on the floor. Grasp the backs of the thighs with your hands. Breathe in.

2. Breathe out, contract your abdominals, tilt your pelvis forward and slowly start to roll back, controlling the move with the abdominal muscles and curving the lower back, as if in a 'C' shape, as you roll. Tuck your chin in to your chest slightly, lengthen along the neck and focus your eyes straight out in front of you.

3. Continue rolling down through the spine, one vertebra at a time, similar to a ball, allowing your feet to come off the floor as you roll, keeping your knees tucked into your chest. Keep your hands in position on your thighs or else your ankles, whichever feels more comfortable.

4. When you reach your furthest point (without rolling any further than onto the shoulders),

WATCH OUT!

This is challenging for some, particularly those with weak abdominals and tightness in the lower back – avoid it until you can do the Rolling back exercise on pages 136–7 with ease. Do not attempt this exercise if you have neck problems.

Benefits
- Strengthens the abdominal core.
- Mobilizes the spine.
- Releases tightness in the lower back.

breathe in and use the abdominals to roll back up to sitting – momentum will help you, but it is the abdominals that control the movement. Keep your knees tucked in towards your chest. Repeat five to ten times.

Option

Once you have mastered this move, try starting from a balanced sitting position with your feet raised, initiating the move from your abdominals instead of pushing off from the floor with your feet.

▼ Depending on your flexibility, you may prefer to hold the outsides of ankles instead of your thighs.

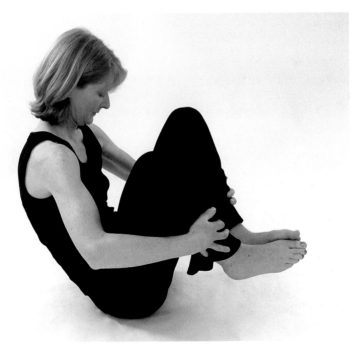

▶ Rocker

**The Rocker is a very demanding exercise and should only
be attempted once the previous moves – Rolling back and
Rolling like a ball – have been completely mastered.**

1. Sit upright with your legs in front of you, slightly
   apart, knees bent and feet flat on the floor.
   Lengthen up through the spine, drop the
   shoulders and draw the shoulderblades down
   into your back. Place your hands around your
   ankles and lift your legs off the floor slightly, one
   at a time, keeping your knees apart and bringing
   your toes together, into a balanced position.

2. Breathe in and lengthen up through the spine
   and neck, then breathe out, contract the
   abdominals, tilt the pelvis forward, and extend
   your legs, keeping the knees soft and the toes
   softly pointed. Extend the legs only as far as
   you can without losing control or balance – it is
   much more important for you to maintain the

▼ Extend your legs only as
far as you can without
losing control or balance.

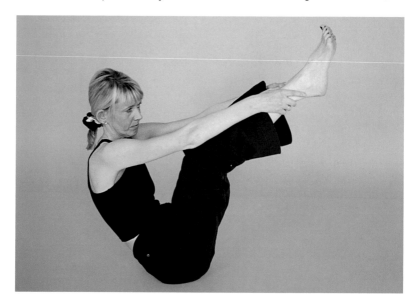

correct position than it is for you to straighten the legs. If it is too difficult for you to hold your ankles, then hold your calves instead.

3. Once you have extended the legs as far as you are able, breathe in, then breathe out, contract the abdominals and lower the legs back down, one at a time. Repeat five times, without touching the floor with your toes if possible.

Option

When you have developed good balance, strength in the abdominals and flexibility in the lower back, you are ready to move on:

1. With the legs extended, exhale, contract the abdominals, tilt the pelvis forward and roll down through the spine, vertebra by vertebra, in a smooth movement. Keep the spine lengthened. Look forward for balance.

2. Continue rolling back, taking your legs over your head – the legs should be straight, if possible with the knees soft. When you have reached your furthest point, breathe in, then breathe out and rock back to the sitting position, controlling the movement with the abdominals and allowing the momentum of the move to help you. Repeat five to ten times.

WATCH OUT!
- Do not attempt this exercise until you have fully mastered Rolling like a ball (pages 138–9).
- If this exercise is too challenging for you, practise Rolling back (pages 136–7) and Rolling like a ball (pages 138–9) to improve spinal strength and flexibility.
- Avoid this exercise if you have any neck problems.

MUST KNOW

Benefits
- Mobilizes the spine.
- Builds strength in the abdominal area and legs.
- Stretches the hamstrings.
- Improves balance and stability.

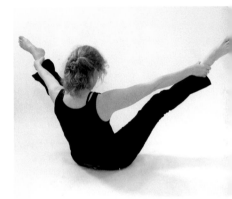

▲ With practice and good balance, the move can be achieved with straight legs.

Opposite arm & leg stretch

When you perform this stretch, try not to raise the legs or arms too high. Keep them level with the hips and shoulders – think of lengthening away from you rather than lifting them.

1. Position yourself on all fours, with hands beneath your shoulders and knees directly beneath your hips.

2. Drop your shoulders down away from your ears and pull your shoulderblades down into your back.

3. Breathe in and lengthen along the spine and neck, focusing your eyes straight down to the floor.

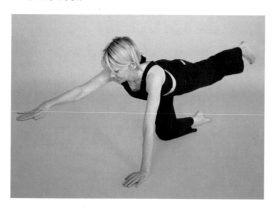

◀ Make sure your hips remain stable as you extend the legs and arms.

MUST KNOW

Benefits
• Improves strength and stability.
• Improves posture and balance.
• Tones the legs, buttocks and hips.
• Stretches the spine.

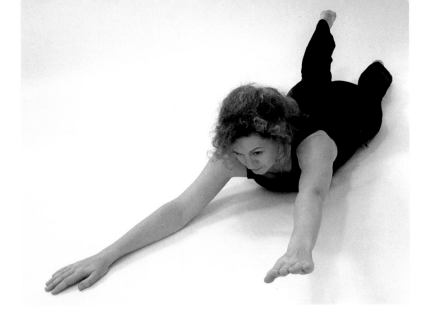

▲ If you do not have good enough balance or control to perform this exercise, practise the movement with your body stretched out flat on the floor (see also Horizontal star, page 114).

4. Breathe out, contract the abdominals and lengthen the right arm and left leg, sliding them away from you, then raising them off the ground to approximately the same level as the hips and shoulders, keeping the elbows soft as you lengthen and making sure that the arms and legs stay in line with the body.

5. Breathe in and release back down. Repeat for the other arm and leg. Do the sequence five to ten times, using opposite arms and legs each time and alternating with each repetition.

Option 1

If you have difficulty balancing, try lifting the limbs one at a time (right arm, then left leg, then left arm, then right leg), until your balance improves.

Option 2

To increase the intensity of the movement, try holding the extended position (with one arm and one leg raised), breathe in, then breathe out, contract the abdominals and lower the arm and leg back down to the starting position.

Shoulder stretch

This is great for stretching not only the shoulders but also the upper back. Use a smooth movement throughout as you stretch the arm forward and bring it back to the starting position.

1. Carefully kneel on the floor on all fours, with your knees directly below your hips and your hands directly beneath your shoulders. Evenly distribute your weight over both your knees. Lengthen along the

▼ Keep the feet on the ground throughout, with the knees and feet in parallel.

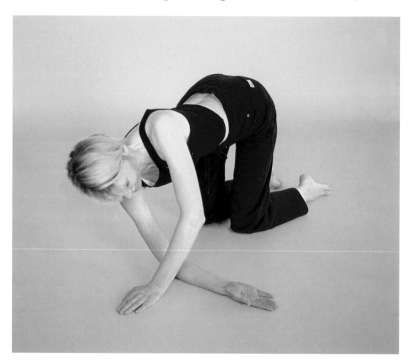

WATCH OUT!

Do not attempt this exercise if you suffer from any knee complaints or have sustained any injury to the knees. Seek medical advice if you are in any doubt.

Benefits

- Stretches the upper back and across the shoulders.
- Releases tension in the upper back.
- Creates a gentle stretch in the spine.

spine and neck and focus the eyes down towards the floor.

2. Breathe in and slowly transfer your weight onto your right hand. Lift your left hand and then position it so that it is placed palm upwards with the back of the hand resting on the floor.

3. Breathe out, contract the abdominal muscles and slide the left hand through the gap under your right shoulder, taking the hand through as far as you can, following the movement of the hand with your eyes. You should feel a stretch across the upper back and shoulders. Only take the hand through as far as you can without losing your balance or indeed losing the abdominal control. It is much more important for you to practise this exercise keeping the correct alignment than it is for you to overreach yourself and struggle to keep control.

4. Breathe in and, maintaining the abdominal contraction, draw the arm back to the starting position. Make sure you maintain the abdominal contraction both as you stretch the arm through behind you and as you bring it back again.Repeat three to five times then repeat for the other side.

SITTING & KNEELING

145

Side stretch

Do not worry if you are unable to stretch very far at first with this move. Your flexibility will increase with practice and you will gradually be able to stretch further towards the knee.

1. Sit on the floor, with your legs apart, knees soft and arms stretched out to the sides just below shoulder level. Bend your right knee and bring your right foot in to rest against the inner thigh of the left leg.

2. Breathe in and lengthen up through the spine and neck.

3. Breathe out, contract the abdominal muscles and raise the right arm, curving it over your head as you lift up out of your waist and stretch the upper body up and over towards the left knee (try to imagine you were stretching over a large beach ball). If you find it difficult to keep the extended leg straight at first, bend the knees slightly.

▼ Keep lengthening up through the spine and along the back of the neck throughout this movement.

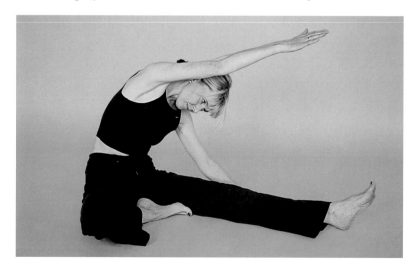

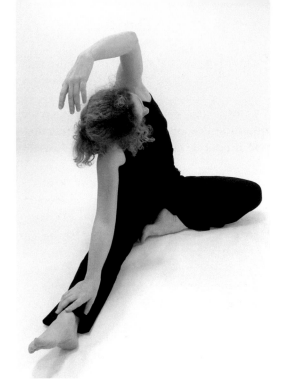

▶ With each repetition, try to increase the stretch, reaching lower down the extended leg every time.

4. Hold the position and breathe in, then breathe out and increase the stretch.

5. Breathe in and release the arm and bring the body back to centre. Repeat the stretch five times, trying to increase the stretch with each repetition, then change your leg position and repeat the entire sequence for the other side.

MUST KNOW

Benefits
- Stretches and tones the waist.
- Stretches and strengthens the legs.
- Improves flexibility.
- Releases tension and tightness in the hamstrings and the lower back.
- Mobilizes the spine.

Tricep dip

This is an excellent upper body strength-building exercise, which works on muscle control for the arms, abdominal core and the legs, as well as improving breath control.

1. Position yourself about 45cm (18in) in front of a sturdy chair, facing away from it. Place your feet hip-width apart, in parallel, toes pointing forwards.

2. Grasp hold of the front corners of the seat and adjust your feet so that your ankles are

▼ Keep the shoulders directly above the hips throughout this exercise.

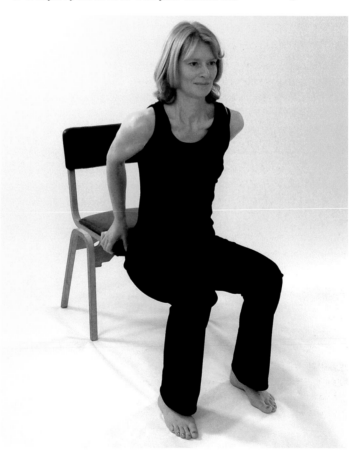

directly below your knees, with your knees at right-angles, thighs parallel to the floor.

3. Breathe in and lengthen along the spine and neck, drop the shoulders and draw the shoulderblades down into your back. Keep your arms straight and elbows soft. Focus your eyes straight in front of you.

4. Breathe out, contract the abdominals, bend your elbows and slowly lower your tailbone to the floor, making sure your that your spine and neck remain in a line, with your hips directly below your shoulders. Lower yourself as far as you are able while keeping the abdominal contraction and maintaining control. Do not lower all the way to the floor – this strength-building exercise should be a slow, controlled, continuous motion, so keep the tailbone a few inches (2–5cm) from the floor.

5. When you have reached your furthest position, breathe in as you raise yourself back up to the 'sitting' position once again. Repeat three to five times.

Option

Try the same exercise with the knees and ankles together, squeezing the inner thighs and the buttocks as you lower and raise.

WATCH OUT!

Avoid this exercise if you have wrist or shoulder problems.

MUST KNOW

Benefits
- Strengthens and stretches the arm muscles.
- Improves posture and alignment.
- Develops muscle control.
- Strengthens the abdominal core and the leg muscles.
- Improves breath control.

▶ Hip flexor stretch

This stretch is designed to gently increase the flexibility in your hips and release tension by lengthening the hip flexor muscles to give you a wider range of motion.

1. Stand with your feet apart. Bend the knees and place your hands on the floor. Step back with the right foot, extending the leg back as far as you can, then lowering the knee to the floor, making sure that the knee and foot are in line with the right hip.

MUST KNOW

Benefits
- Strengthens and stretches the hip flexor muscles, the hamstrings, the quadriceps and the gluteals.
- Improves balance.
- Releases tightness in the pelvic area.

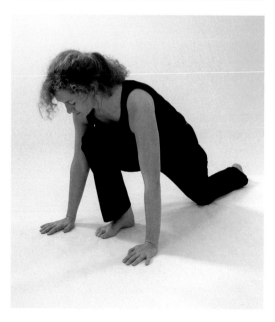

◀ Make sure that the knee and foot of the extended leg are in line with the hip.

► Keep the body facing forwards – avoid twisting to one side or the other as you stretch.

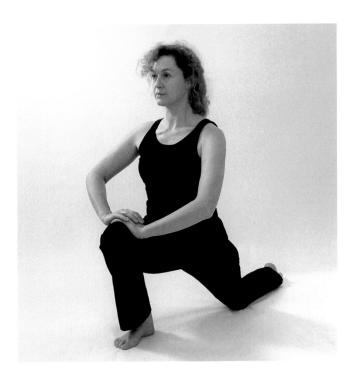

2. Breathe in and bring the hands up to rest on the left knee.

3. Exhale, contract the abdominals, and lengthen the body forward over the left knee, to create a stretch through the front of the left thigh. Keep the lengthening up through the spine and neck as you stretch. Breathe in and release. Repeat the stretch five to ten times, breathing out as you stretch forward and in as you release. Repeat for the other leg.

4. To increase the stretch still further, breathe in, tuck the toes of the right foot under and raise the right knee up away from the floor. Exhale as you lengthen the body forward over the left knee increase the stretch. Inhale and release. Repeat this stretch five to ten times. Repeat for the other side.

▶ Glut stretch

Gluteal muscles are key for people who suffer from stiffness in the lower back. This stretch will improve the effectiveness of these muscles in providing stability to the lumbar area.

1. Lie on your back with your legs bent, knees pointing to the ceiling and your arms by your sides. Breathe in and float the legs up, one at a time, towards the chest. Cross the right

---

MUST KNOW

Benefits
- Stretches the gluteal muscles and the lower back.
- Reduces tightness and stiffness in the lower back.
- Improves flexibility.

▼ Keep the upper body, neck and shoulders as relaxed as possible throughout this stretch.

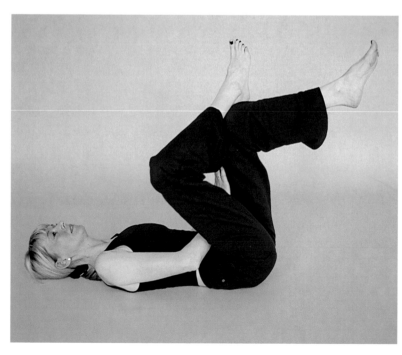

If you feel any pain in your lower back, stop and release the legs a little – you may be trying to work too hard for your current level of ability. If the discomfort continues, stop and, if necessary, seek medical advice.

▼ Hold the stretch for five to ten breaths, drawing the leg closer to the chest on every out breath.

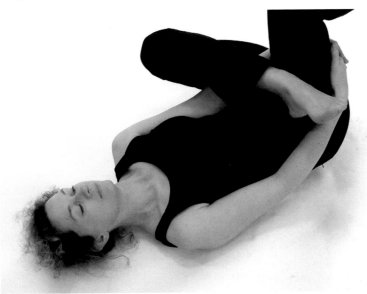

ankle over the left knee. Place the hands around the left thigh. Lengthen along the spine and back of your neck and focus your eyes up to the ceiling.

MUST KNOW

Muscles should always be stretched out after you have finished any sequence of strengthening exercises.

2. Breathe out, contract the abdominals, and pull your left thigh gently in towards the body, stretching the muscles in the right thigh. Hold this stretch for five to ten breaths, drawing the leg closer to the chest each time you breathe out. Breathe in and release the legs back to the starting position.

3. Repeat on the other side.

SITTING & KNEELING

153

Foot exercises

Your feet carry the whole weight of your body throughout the day and so should not be ignored when it comes to exercise. Look after your feet and they will look after you.

Lifting the arches

1. Place your feet on the floor in parallel and extend the toes.
2. Draw the toes slowly back along the floor towards you, lifting the arches.
3. Release the arches and lengthen the toes. Repeat ten times.

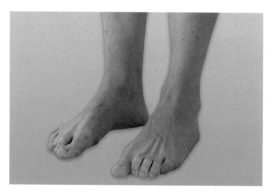

◄ Draw your toes slowly back along the floor towards you, lifting the arches of the feet.

▼ Flex the toes up as far as you can, keeping the rest of the foot on the floor.

Toe flexes

1. Place your feet on the floor in parallel and extend the toes.
2. Flex the toes up as far as you can, keeping the rest of the foot in contact with the floor.
3. Release and extend the toes. Repeat the flexes ten times.

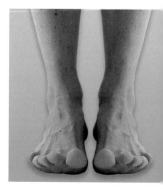

MUST KNOW

Benefits
• Strengthens and mobilizes the feet and ankles.
• Improves circulation to the legs.

Toe teaser

1. Place your feet on the floor in parallel and extend the toes, spreading them as wide as you can.
2. Lift the big toes, leaving the other toes on the floor.
3. Switch and place the big toes on the floor as you lift the rest of the toes. Repeat ten times.
4. Now, try lifting each toe in turn, starting with the big toe, then releasing it back to the floor and lifting the next toe, and so on. Repeat five to ten times. If you cannot manage this at first, use your hands to lift each toe.

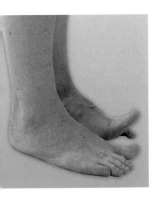

▲ With your feet on the floor, lift your big toes, leaving the other toes on the ground.

MUST KNOW

- These exercises can be done at any time and only take a few minutes – either standing or sitting, whichever is most convenient.
- Keep your breathing slow and even.
- Do not roll the feet in to the centre or out to the sides.

Marching feet

1. Place your feet on the floor, ankles together, and extend the toes.
2. Raise the ball of one foot, keeping the heel on the ground.
3. Roll down through the foot, placing the ball of the foot on the ground and slowly raising the heel.
4. Repeat five times, then switch and repeat for the other foot.
5. Lift the toes of your right foot as you lift the heel of the left.
6. Roll down through the feet, raising the heel of your right foot as you lift the toes of your left in a 'marching' motion.
7. Repeat ten times.

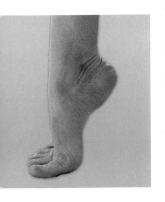

▲ Raise the heel of your right foot as you perform 'marching feet' with the toes of your left foot.

Spinal twist

When you perform this exercise, sit upright, with your shoulders directly above your hips and try to avoid leaning back as you twist round.

1. Sit on the floor with your knees raised, feet on the floor. Tuck your right foot under your left hip and bring your left foot around, placing it next to your right thigh, with your left foot pointing forwards.

2. Start to twist your upper body around to the right slightly and place your left arm along the

◀ Do not take the head any further than the shoulders as you twist and stretch.

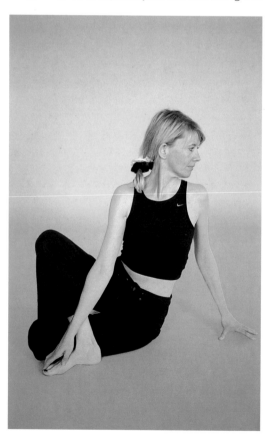

Benefits
- Stretches and strengthens the spine.
- Releases neck, shoulder and lower-back tension.
- Stretches the muscles of the hips and buttocks.

inside of your left calf. Avoid letting your weight sink into the floor – keep lifting through the waist, up and out of the hips. Breathe in.

3. Breathe out, contract the abdominals and twist around to the right with your shoulders and upper body, looking over your right shoulder and placing the fingertips of your right hand on the floor, slightly behind you, to steady you. Stay sitting upright, directing the crown of your head up to the ceiling – do not lean back. Keep your shoulders dropped and your shoulderblades drawn down into your back. Press with the left arm against the inside of the left thigh to help you twist. Hold this position for a count of five, then breathe in and release – repeat three to five times in total, breathing out as you twist and stretch and breathing in as you release back to centre.

4. Switch positions, tucking your left foot under your right hip, placing your right foot next to your left thigh, your right arm against your right inner thigh and then placing the fingertips of your left hand on the floor to steady you as you twist and stretch around to the left, this time looking over your left shoulder. Repeat the stretch three to five times on this side.

SITTING & KNEELING

157

The Cat

This exercise is one of the gentlest and simplest ways to stretch out the back. If you wake up with a stiff back or neck, spend a couple of minutes doing cat stretches.

1. Kneel on all fours with your knees positioned directly below your hips, and your hands directly below your shoulders, with your fingers pointing forward away from the body. The feet should rest on the ground in line with the hips and shoulders, toes pointing away from the body. Keep the arms straight and the elbows soft. Breathe in and lengthen along the spine and the back of the neck.

WATCH OUT!

Beware of over-arching as you release down, as this can cause pressure in the lower back.

2. Breathe out, contract the abdominals, tuck the pelvis under, and drop your chin to your chest, lengthening through the back of the neck. As you continue to breathe out, arch the upper back towards the ceiling, like a cat, stretching

▼ Contract the abdominal muscles, tuck the pelvis under and drop your chin to your chest.

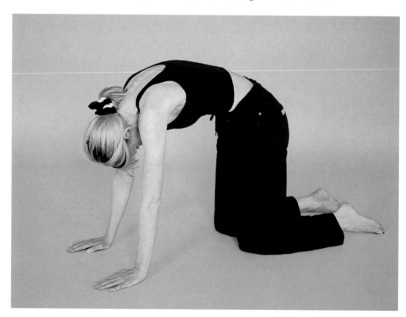

Benefits
- Relieves tension in the back and shoulders.
- Improves posture.
- Stretches the chest and shoulders.
- Strengthens the arms.

the entire length of the spine. Keep the hips and shoulders level.

3. Breathe in and release back to centre; then reverse the curve slightly, lifting the tailbone to the ceiling and flattening out at the waist. Do not drop down too far; this part of the move is a release rather than a stretch. Lift the head so the neck is in line with the spine and lengthen along the spine. Repeat five to ten times, breathing out as you arch upwards and in as you release the spine back down. Use a continuous movement, in time with the breathing.

▼ Release the move back to the centre and, very slightly, reverse the curve in the spine – do not drop too far.

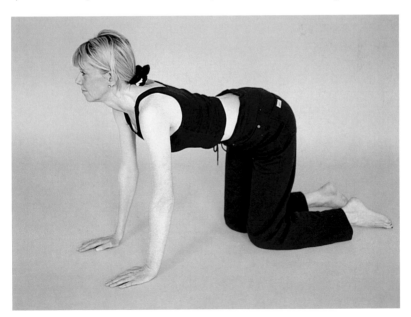

Rest position

This position can be used to relax at the end of a Pilates session or during a workout if your back and neck becomes tense and stiff.

1. Kneel on all fours, with your knees below your hips and your hands below your shoulders, fingers pointing forward. Breathe in and lengthen along the spine and back of the neck.

> **WATCH OUT!**
>
> This move should be avoided by anyone suffering from knee problems.

2. Breathe out, contracting the abdominals, and lower your body back until you are sitting on your heels with your chest resting on the front of your thighs. Stretch your arms out in front of you in line with your shoulders.

3. Breathe in and relax your forehead down to the floor. Do not hunch the shoulders – keep them dropped down, away from the ears.

4. Hold this position for five to ten breaths, allowing the spine to stretch and the body to relax a little more with every outbreath. Breathe in and come back up to centre.

▼ Don't worry if you cannot sit right back on your heels at first – your hips and spine will gradually become more flexible.

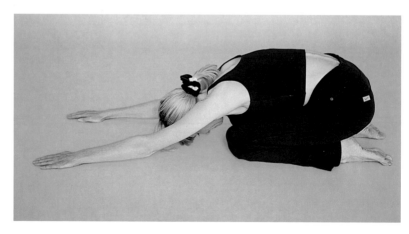

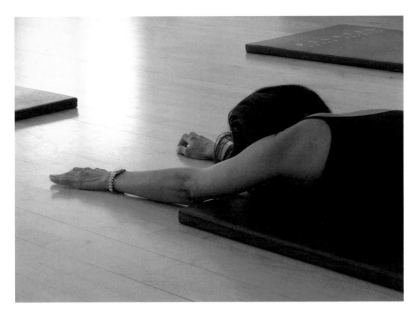

▲ Lying at full stretch, with your entire body on the floor, can be an option if you suffer from severe knee problems.

MUST KNOW

Benefits

- Gently stretches the spine.
- Releases tension in the back and neck.
- Improves circulation.

Option

This exercise is the same as discussed on page 160, except for the arm position. Experiment to find out which of the two positions suits you best. If you suffer from tension or stiffness in the neck and shoulders, you may find that this position is more comfortable for you.

1. As you sit back on your heels, slide your arms back along the floor and place them close to your sides, palms facing upwards. Lengthen down through the arms, taking the hands back as far as you can, then relax the arms and shoulders as you bring the forehead down to the floor.

want to know more?

Take it to the next level...

Go to...
▶ **The neutral position** – page 30
▶ **Chest stretch** – page 176

Have a go...
▶ **T'ai chi, yoga and yogalates**
many Pilates enthusiasts also enjoy yoga or t'ai chi classes, as well as yogalates – a fun combination of yoga and Pilates moves
▶ **Exercise to music**
can improve your mood, and may also boost your brain power

Other sources
▶ **Articles on fitness and health topics**
try websites like www.discoverfitness.com

on the

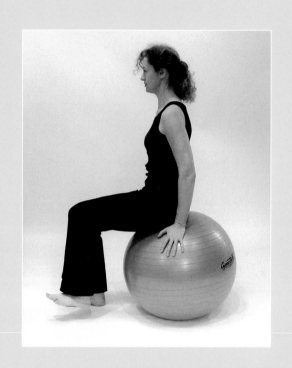

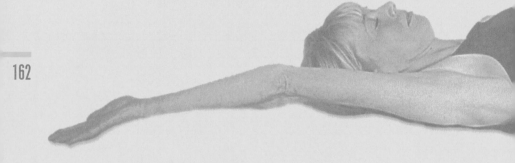

ball

Exercising on a ball encourages you to work your abdominal muscles, strengthening your central core and improving your posture, balance, alignment and co-ordination as you move. Certain moves will increase flexibility, while others demand more strength than if they were performed on a flat surface.

▶ Warm-ups

When choosing a ball, the basic guideline is that, when sitting on the ball, your knees should form an angle of no less than 90 degrees, with your thighs roughly parallel to the floor.

Bounces and circles

1. Sit comfortably on the ball with your feet hip-width apart, your ankles directly below your knees and your weight evenly distributed over both feet. Rest your hands either on your thighs or by your sides on the ball.

2. Bounce gently up and down a few times, keeping your feet in contact with the floor and making sure that the ball stays in position, without rolling forwards or backwards or side to side.

3. Keeping your feet in contact with the floor and your upper body in position, contract your abdominals and gently circle your hips three times to the right then three times to the left, allowing the ball to roll under you slightly as you do so and making sure that the movement is smooth and controlled throughout. Repeat three to five times.

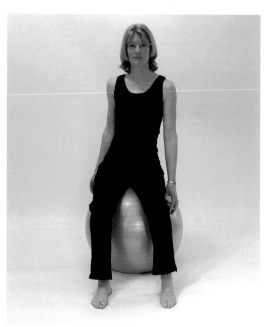

◀ Keeping your feet in contact with the floor, circle your hips, allowing the ball to roll under you slightly.

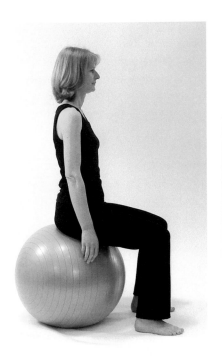

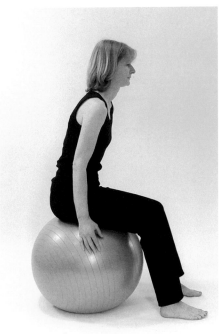

▲ Roll the ball backwards very slightly, allowing your lower back to arch a little.

▲ Roll the ball forwards, rounding your lower back slightly.

Forward and back

1. Sit on the ball with your feet in parallel, hip-width apart. Lengthen up through the spine and along the back of the neck. Focus your eyes straight ahead and check that your spine is in the neutral position. Breathe in, contract the abdominals and breathe out as you roll the ball backwards very slightly, allowing your lower back to arch a little, but all the time making sure that you keep contracting the abdominals as you move.

2. Breathe in and come back to centre, then breathe out and roll the ball forwards slightly, rounding your lower back slightly as you move. Breathe in and come back to centre.

3. Repeat three to five times, making sure that the abdominals stay contracted throughout and checking that your spine is in neutral each time that you return to centre.

Foot lifts

This move is more difficult than it appears, as the ball is not a stable surface and a great deal of control is required to keep your pelvis level and maintain your balance without wobbling or leaning to one side.

1. Sit comfortably on the ball with your feet slightly more than hip-width apart, your ankles directly below your knees. Rest your hands either on your thighs or by your sides on the ball.

2. Breathe in, lengthen up through the spine and along the back of the neck, contract the abdominals and lift one foot up away from the floor an inch or two (2–5cm), keeping your knee at right angles. Breathe in and lower. Try not to change your position or alignment as you raise the foot and lower the foot. Repeat for the other side. Repeat the sequence three to five times.

◀ When you raise one foot from the floor, focus on contracting the abdominals to remain stable on the ball.

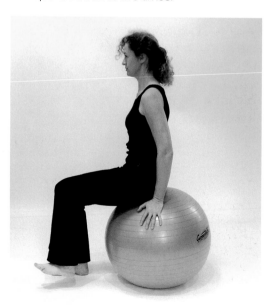

Rolling the ball

1. Lie on your back with your spine in neutral and your feet flat on the ball, your arms resting by your sides. Breathe in, contract the abdominals, then breathe out and extend your legs, pushing the ball away from you, but making sure that your spine remains in neutral.

2. Breathe in and return to the start position. Repeat three to five times.

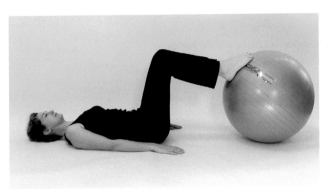

◀ Keeping your spine in neutral, breathe out and extend your legs, pushing the ball away from you.

Hip rolls

1. Lie on your back with your spine in neutral and your calves resting on the ball with your knees at right angles. Place your arms by your sides. Breathe in, contract the abdominals then breathe out and roll the knees over to the right, letting the left hip raise up slightly as you roll, but making sure that the abdominals stay contracted and that the movement remains slow and controlled throughout.

2. Breathe in and return to centre, then repeat for the other side. Repeat the sequence three to five times on each side.

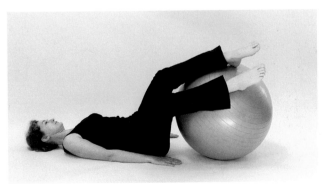

◀ As you gently roll, contract the abdominals and keep the movement slow and controlled.

▶ Abdominals

Moves using the ball demand more strength and control than if they were performed on a flat, stable surface. The exercises on the following pages will really improve strength.

Spine curls

Make sure that you have mastered the basic level before you move on to the more advanced position – only take the movement as far as you can while maintaining control of the ball and keeping the abdominal contraction.

1. Lie on your back with your spine in the neutral position and your calves resting on the ball with your knees at right angles. Place your arms by your sides. Lengthen along the spine and the back of the neck. Breathe in, contract the abdominals then breathe out, squeeze the buttocks and tilt the pelvis upwards slightly, slowly raising the tailbone away from the floor by no more than an inch (2–3cm). Breathe in and release. Repeat five to ten times.

> **MUST KNOW**
>
> **Benefits**
> • Increases flexibility in the spine.
> • Strengthens the abdominal muscles.
> • Improves co-ordination and control.

▼ Gradually peel the spine away from the floor a little more with each repetition.

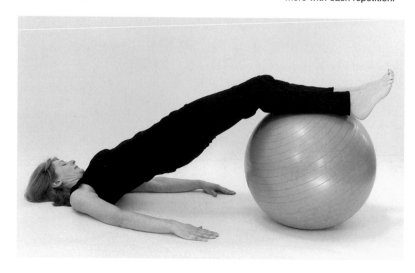

2. Repeat the above sequence several times, but this time lifting the tailbone a little more with each repetition, gradually curling the spine up away from the floor, one vertebra at a time. Breathe out and roll slowly back down through the spine.

Option 1

Breathe in, contract the abdominals, then breathe out and roll all the way up through the spine, starting with the tailbone, until you are resting on your shoulders with your body in a diagonal slope, your spine in neutral. Breathe in, then breathe out and take the arms back behind the head. Breathe in and release the arms then roll slowly back down through the spine. Repeat three to five times.

Option 2

Repeat the above step, this time keeping your arms in position above the head as you release the spine back down to the floor, then breathing in as you bring the arms back to your sides. Repeat this step three to five times.

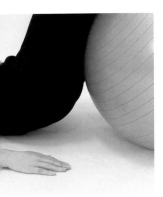

▲ In the basic level of the exercise, only raise your tailbone a little way from the floor.

▼ A more advanced move involves taking your arms back behind the head as you release the spine back down.

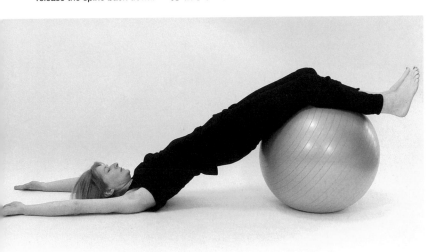

The Hundred

Make sure that your weight remains evenly balanced over both feet throughout this exercise.

Keep the abdominals contracted throughout and the pelvis lifted, so that the body remains in line with the thighs.

1. Sit upright on the ball with your feet flat on the floor and your hands resting by your sides.

2. Breathe in, contract the abdominals and tilt the pelvis upwards slightly towards the ceiling, then breathe out and slowly walk your feet away from you, rolling down until your head and shoulders are resting on the ball, your arms still at your sides.

3. Lengthen your arms away from you and lift and lower your hands in a pulsing action, breathing in to a count of five and then out to a count of five. Continue until you reach a total of 100.

4. Breathe in and roll slowly back up to sitting position.

MUST KNOW

Benefits
- Strengthens the abdominals.
- Works the backs of the legs and the gluteals.
- Improves balance and stability.

▼ Slowly walk your feet until your head and shoulders are resting on the ball, with your arms parallel to the floor.

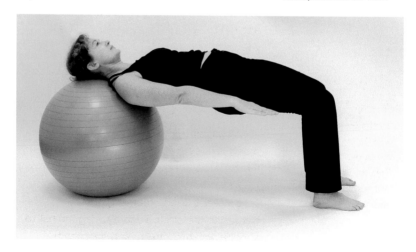

ON THE BALL

170

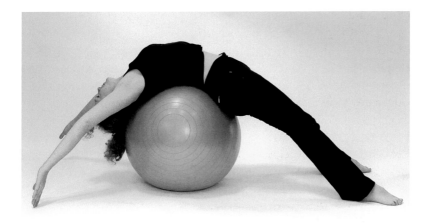

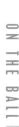
▲ Allow the ball to completely support you as you breathe out, stretching your arms and legs away from you to increase the stretch along the front of the body.

Abdominal stretch

Check that you are positioned so that you are lying comfortably with your back supported by the ball. Keep lengthening along the back of the neck as you stretch.

1. Sit upright on the ball with your feet on the floor a little more than hip-width apart.

2. Slowly walk your feet away from you, rolling down onto the ball until you are positioned with your legs outstretched and the ball supporting your back. Relax your head, neck and shoulders down onto the ball. Let your arms relax out to the sides.

3. Breathe in, then breathe out as you extend your legs away from you, allowing gravity to create a stretch across the chest and down the front of the body.

4. Take several deep breaths, gradually increasing the stretch and allowing the ball to support you more with each out breath.

MUST KNOW

Benefits
- Stretches the chest and the front of the body.
- Releases tension in the spine, neck and shoulders.

171

▶ The back

Using a ball is an excellent way to increase your range of movement, particularly the flexibility in your back. Strength in the back is also improved in a gentle and safe way.

Horizontal star

Check that your back remains level throughout and focus on lengthening your neck.

If it is too difficult for you to maintain your balance as you raise both one arm and one leg, practise raising only one limb at a time until your strength and stability have improved.

1. Position yourself so that you are lying on your front with the ball under your stomach to support you.

MUST KNOW

Benefits
• Strengthens the back.
• Improves balance, posture, muscle control and co-ordination.

WATCH OUT!

Keep your abdominals contracted as you stretch, to help support your lower back.

Do not raise the arms and legs too high – concentrate on lengthening them away from your body as you lift.

▼ Keep your abdominals contracted to steady you as you raise the opposite arm and leg.

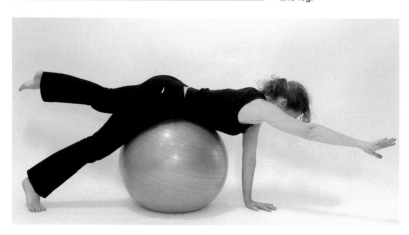

2. Breathe in, contract your abdominals and breath out as you raise your right arm and your right leg, lengthening them away from you.

3. Breathe in and lower. Repeat for the opposite arm and leg, then, alternating the arms and legs, repeat the sequence five to ten times.

Spine stretch

Relax your neck and shoulders and drop your head as you allow gravity to stretch through your spine.

1. Position yourself face down so that the ball is under your waist, supporting the weight of your body. Your toes should be touching the floor on one side of the ball and your hands (or forearms, if that is more comfortable) resting on the floor on the other.

MUST KNOW

Benefits
- Gently stretches the back.
- Releases tension along the spine and in the lower back.

2. Take several deep breaths, allowing your body to relax a little more, and the stretch to increase, with each out breath.

▼ Keep your toes on the floor and allow the ball to support your weight as you lean forward onto the floor.

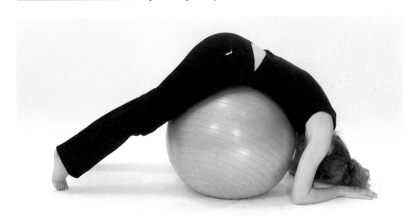

The legs

These exercises are ideal for strengthening the leg
and buttock muscles, as well as improving posture,
balance and all-over muscle control.

Squats against the wall

Make sure that your weight is evenly balanced
over both of your feet throughout this exercise
and that your hips, knees and feet stay in
alignment.

Keep your arms relaxed and your shoulders
dropped down away from your ears.

Feel your back rolling over the ball in a
smooth, controlled movement as you raise and
lower yourself.

1. Stand against a wall with the ball resting in the
   small of your back, your feet in parallel hip-
   width apart, arms by your side.

2. Lean your weight back into the ball slightly,
   inhale and contract your abdominals. Breathe
   out and bend your knees, lowering yourself
   into a squat position with your knees at an
   angle of 90 degrees.

3. Breathe in, keeping the abdominals
   contracted, then breathe out and slowly
   come back up to standing. Repeat the
   sequence five to ten times.

WATCH OUT!

Do not lower yourself too far down, as this could
put unnecessary strain on the knee joints. Aim to
lower yourself only until your knees are at a 90-
degree angle, with your thighs parallel to the floor.

MUST KNOW

Benefits
• Strengthens the leg
  muscles.
• Improves posture
  and muscle control.

▼ Lower yourself into a
squat position against the
ball, knees at 90 degrees,
shoulders relaxed.

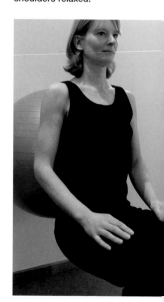

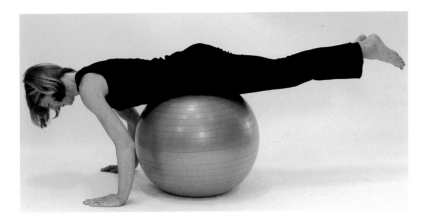

Leg lifts

Keep the back and neck lengthened, the pelvis level and the abdominals contracted as you lift and lower the legs. The movement should be slow and controlled throughout.

1. Position yourself so that you are on your hands and knees with the ball placed under your stomach, with your weight resting on the ball. Straighten your knees so that you bring yourself up onto your toes.

2. Breathe in, contract your abdominals and breath out as you extend your right leg, lengthening along the spine and back of the neck as you raise the leg up away from the floor.

3. Breathe in and lower, then repeat for the opposite leg. Repeat the entire sequence five to ten times, using alternate legs.

Option

Bring your weight forward slightly onto your hands, contract the abdominals, then breathe out and slowly raise both legs together. Breathe in and slowly lower back down. Repeat five times.

MUST KNOW

Benefits
- Strengthens and tones the leg and buttock muscles.
- Improves balance and muscle control.
- Builds strength and stamina.

ON THE BALL

175

▶ The upper body

The arms, shoulder muscles and upper body are all given a good workout with these exercises. Avoid the chest stretch if you suffer from any knee problems though.

Chest stretch

Do not drop at the waist as you stretch the shoulder downwards. Keep your spine in neutral and your neck lengthened.

1. Position yourself on all fours with the ball at your right side. Place your right arm on the ball with your fingers pointing forwards and your elbow at a right angle, upper arm in line with the shoulder joint.

2. Breathe in, contract the abdominals; breathe out and lower your right shoulder towards the floor slightly, rotating your head to the left.

3. Breathe in and come back up to centre; roll the ball to the left and repeat for the other side.

4. Repeat the sequence three to five times on each side.

MUST KNOW

Benefits
- Increases strength and stamina.
- Strengthens the arms and upper body.
- Improves balance and co-ordination.

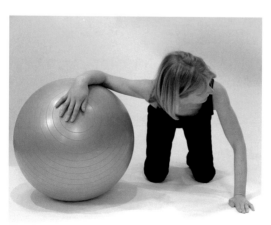

◀ As you lower your right shoulder, rotate your head to the left.

Press ups

Keep the back and neck lengthened as you raise and lower the upper body. Make sure that your abdominals are contracted and that your body remains in alignment throughout this sequence – particularly during the more advanced variations.

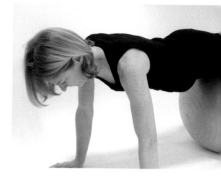

▲ To increase the difficulty, walk forwards on your hands so that the ball supports your thighs.

1. Position yourself so that you are on your hands and knees with the ball placed under your stomach, your weight resting on the ball. Walk forwards on your hands until the ball supports your hips and your feet are raised up away from the floor. (If you find this too difficult, take the ball back so that your toes are touching the floor.)

2. Breathe in, contract your abdominals and breath out as you bend your elbows and slowly lower your upper body down towards the floor. Breathe in and raise back up to centre. Repeat five to ten times.

Option

Once you have mastered the above steps, increase the difficulty by walking further forwards on your hands so that the ball is supporting first your thighs, then your shins and finally, most difficult of all, your ankles.

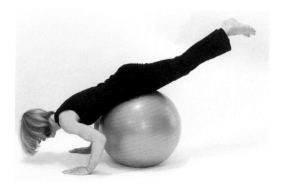

▲ With the ball supporting your hips, bend your elbows and lower your upper body down towards the floor.

want to know more?

Take it to the next level...

Go to...
▶ Pilates for you – pages 18–19
▶ Pilates for a healthy body – pages 22–3

Have a go...
▶ Physio balls and other equipment
including foam rollers, balance trainers, core boards and more are fun. Visit www.physicalcompany.co.uk
▶ Pilates studio classes
for some online studio exercises, visit www.bodyzone.com

Other sources
▶ Publications
visit www.amazon.com for more books

pilates

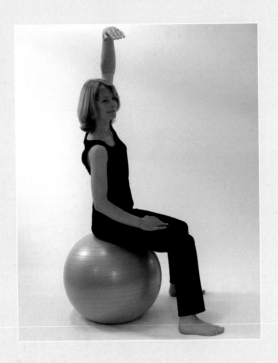

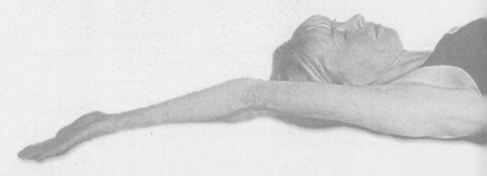

routines

Pilates exercises are designed to develop muscles uniformly and so it is important that a balanced series of movements are performed during a workout. Warming up the muscles is the most important part of any routine and should on no account be missed before any workout.

▶ Suggested routines

Routines need to be realistic – if you are short of time, do not set yourself dozens of exercises to do, as you will inevitably rush through them and not reap the full benefits.

Short daily routines

If you choose to do short daily routines, you will find that once you have warmed up each day, you will not have much time to work intensively with many of the exercises. But it is better to choose fewer moves and work in a focussed, controlled manner than to rush through a large number of moves and risk practising them incorrectly. Vary your daily programme so that, within the course of a week, you have included some exercises for all the different areas of the body.

Here are seven suggestions to get you started; page numbers follow for ease of use.

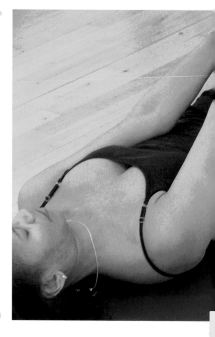

▼ Make sure that you include exercises for all the different muscle groups in your Pilates routine.

SHORT DAILY ROUTINE 1

Breathing *34*
Rolling down the wall *35*
Arm swings *37*
Shoulder hunches *39*
Alternate hip openings *40*
Arm raises *50*
Waist twist *52*
Push up *56*
Hundred *66*
Neck pull *68*
One-leg circles *78*
Pillow squeeze 1 *110*
Horizontal star *114*
Rolling back *136*
Arm and leg stretch *142*
Cat *158*
Rest position *160*

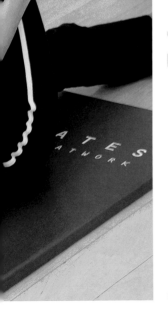

SHORT DAILY ROUTINE 2

Breathing 34
Rolling down the wall 35
Standing balance 36
Arm raises into arm
   circles 38
Alternate hip openings 40
Hip folds 42
Egyptian arm circles 44
Spine curls 60
Hundred 66
Neck stretch 70

Single-leg stretch 72
Double-leg
   stretch 74
Shoulder lifts 80
Arm openings 82
Arm circles 62
Chest opener 54
Spine stretch 132
Shoulder stretch 144
Rest position 160

SHORT DAILY ROUTINE 3

Breathing 34
Rolling down the wall 35
Arm swings 37
Arm raises into arm
circles 38
Alternate hip openings 40
Hip folds 42
Egyptian arm circles 44
Arm raises 48
Push up 56

Hip rolls 64
Hundred 66
Windmill 84
Leg lifts 96
Double leg lifts
   (side) 102
Swan position 124
Pillow squeeze 2 129
Spinal twist 156
Rest position 160

SHORT DAILY ROUTINE 4

Breathing 34
Standing balance 36
Arm raises into arm
   circles 38
Shoulder hunches 39
Egyptian arm
   circles 44
Arm raises 48
Hip rolls 64
Hundred 66
Neck pull 68
Neck stretch 70
Single-leg stretch 72

Double-leg
   stretch 74
Hamstring stretch 76
Inner thigh
   stretch 104
Horizontal star 114
Spine stretch 132
Spine twist 134
Rolling like a ball 138
Hip flexor stretch 150
Glut stretch 152
Foot exercises 154

SHORT DAILY ROUTINE 5

Breathing *34*
Rolling down the wall *35*
Arm swings *37*
Shoulder hunches *39*
Alternate hip
  openings *40*
Hip folds *42*
Hip rolls *64*
Hundred *66*
Push up *56*
Neck pull *68*
Double-leg stretch *74*
Corkscrew *86*
Rocker *140*

Jack knife *88*
Rolling up *94*
Ankle circles *108*
Pillow squeeze 1 *110*
One-leg heel
  kicks *118*
Shoulder press *115*
Dart *117*
Leg pull *120*
Arm and leg
  stretch *142*
Cat *158*
Rest position *160*

SHORT DAILY ROUTINE 6

Breathing *34*
Rolling down the wall *35*
Arm raises into arm circles *38*
Shoulder hunches *39*
Alternate hip openings *40*
Push up *56*
Spine curls *60*
Hip rolls *64*
Hundred *66*
Single-leg stretch *72*
One-leg circles *78*
Teaser *90*
Scissors *92*
Rolling over *106*
Pillow squeeze 1 *110*
Shoulder press *115*
Plank *122*
Side bend *126*
Tricep dip *148*
Arm and leg stretch *142*
Shoulder stretch *144*
Hip flexor stretch *150*

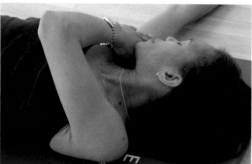

◀ Concentrate on your breathing throughout all your routines and relax into the moves as much as possible.

SHORT DAILY ROUTINE 7

Breathing *34*
Standing balance *36*
Bounces and circles
  (on the ball) *164*
Forward and back
  (on the ball) *165*
Foot lifts (on the ball) *166*
Hip rolls (on the ball) *167*
Spine curls
  (on the ball) *169*
Hundred (on the ball) *170*

Squats against the
  wall (on the ball) *174*
Abdominal stretch
  (on the ball) *171*
Press ups
  (on the ball) *176*
Horizontal star
  (on the ball) *172*
Chest stretch
  (on the ball) *177*

Two to three times weekly routines

If you prefer to set aside longer amounts of time to devote to your exercise programme, here are a few suggestions for some longer routines. Again, make sure that you vary your sessions each time, to include some exercises for all the different areas of the body.

2/3 TIMES WEEKLY 1

Breathing *34*

Rolling down the wall *35*

Standing balance *36*

Arm swings *37*

Shoulder hunches *39*

Alternate hip openings *40*

Arms raises *50*

Waist twist *52*

Chest opener *54*

Push up *56*

Spine curls *60*

Hip rolls *64*

Hundred *66*

Neck pull *68*

Neck stretch *70*

One-leg circles *78*

Single-leg stretch *72*

Double-leg stretch *74*

Shoulder lifts *80*

Arm openings *82*

Corkscrew *86*

Teaser *90*

Rolling up *94*

Leg lifts *96*

Ankle circles *108*

Pillow squeeze 1 *110*

Horizontal star *114*

Shoulder press *115*

Dart *117*

Swan position *124*

Spine stretch *132*

Spine twist *134*

Rolling back *136*

Cat *158*

Rest position *160*

▼ Attending a class under the watchful guidance of an instructor can improve your Pilates technique.

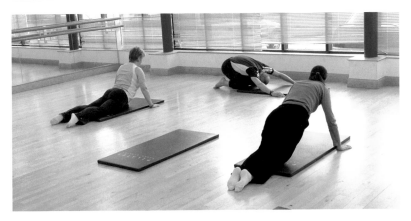

Weekly routines

The following routines are a few suggestions for those people who wish to work at one longer weekly session per week, or for those who have chosen to do two longer sessions per week than the ones given above.

WEEKLY ROUTINE 1

Breathing *26*
Rolling down the wall *35*
Standing balance *36*
Arm swings *37*
Arm raises into arm circles *38*
Shoulder hunches *39*
Alternate hip openings *40*
Hip folds *42*
Egyptian arm circles *44*
Arm raises *50*
Waist twist *52*
Push up *56*
Spine curls *60*

Hip rolls *64*
Hundred *66*
Neck pull *68*
Single-leg stretch *72*
Double-leg stretch *74*
Arm openings *82*
Jack knife *88*
Scissors *92*
Rolling up *94*
Rolling over *106*
Ankle circles *108*
Horizontal star *114*
Arm and leg stretch *142*
Shoulder press *115*
Dart *117*
One-leg heel kicks *118*

Leg pull *120*
Plank *122*
Swan position *124*
Side bend *126*
Spine stretch *132*
Spine twist *134*
Rolling back *136*
Rocker *140*
Side stretch *146*
Hip flexor stretch *150*
Foot exercises *154*
Spinal twist *156*
Cat *158*
Rest position *160*
Pillow squeeze 1 *110*

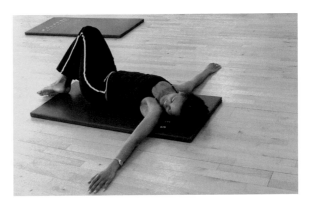

▲ The abdominals are vital in Pilates routines. In this hip roll exercise, the movement should be controlled as you roll and not left to the momentum of your legs to carry you over.

▶ Remember, breathing, posture and warming up are all essential for performing Pilates correctly.

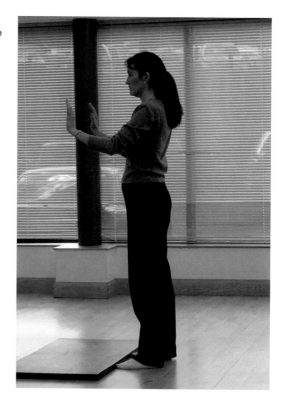

WEEKLY ROUTINE 2

Need to know more?

Useful addresses/Websites

UK

The Body Control Pilates
Association, PO Box 29061,
London WC2H 9TB
www.bodycontrol.co.uk

The Pilates Foundation UK Ltd,
PO Box 36052, London SW16 1XQ
Tel. 07071 781559
www.pilatesfoundation.com

Body Maintenance Studio,
2nd Floor, Pineapple, 7 Langley
Street, London WC2H 9JA

USA

re:Ab Studio, 33 Bleecker Street,
Suite 2C, New York, NY 10012
Tel. (212) 420 9111
www.reabnyc.com

Ultimate Body Control,
30 East 60th Street #606,
New York, NY 10022
www.pilates-ny.com

Pilates Studio of Los Angeles,
8704 Santa Monica Bvd, Suite 300,
West Hollywood, California
Tel. (310) 659 1077
www.pilatestherapy.com

Canada

Moretti Studio, 1115 Sherbrooke
Street West, Montreal, Quebec
Tel. (514) 285 4884
www.pilates-montreal.com

Australia

Body Control Pilates-Australia,
Locked Bag 28/352, Pyrmont
NSW 2009
Tel. (02) 9692 0140
www.info@bodycontrol.co.uk

The Pilates Method Studio, Level 4,
45-56 Holt Street, Surry Hills,
NSW 2010 Tel. (02) 9696 4689
www.pilatesm.com.au

New Zealand

Pilates Exercise Specialists, PO Box
24098, Wellington
Tel. (64) 4 384 1034
www.pilates.nzsites.com

Further reading

*A Pilates' Primer: The Millennium
Edition*, Joseph H. Pilates, William
J. Miller, Bodymind Pub., 2000
Abdominal Training, Christopher M.
Norris, Lyons Press, 2002
Body Control: the Pilates Way,
Lynne Robinson, Pan, 1998
Every Body is Beautiful, Ron
Fletcher, Lippencott, 1978
Everything Pilates, Amy Taylor
Taylor Alpers, Lorna Gentry,
Rachel Taylor Segel, Adams
Media Corporation, 2002
*The Joseph H. Pilates Method at
Home: A Balance, Shape,
Strength, and Fitness Program*,
Eleanor McKenzie, Trevor Blount,
Ulysses Press, 2000

The Official Body Control Fitness Manual, Lynne Robinson, Gordon Thompson, MacMillan, 2002

Pilates, Patricia Lamond, Globe Pequot Press, 2002

The Pilates Body, Brooke Siler, Michael Joseph, 2000

Pilates for a Fabulous Body, Lesley Ackland, Thorsons, 2002

Pilates for Beginners, Kellina Stewart, HarperInformation, 2001

Pilates for Every Body, Denise Austin, Rodale Press, 2002

Pilates Gym, Lynne Robinson and Gerry Convy, Pan, 2001

Pilates on the Ball: The World's Most Popular Workout Using the Exercise Ball, Colleen Craig, Healing Art Press, 2001

The Pilates Powerhouse, Mari Winsor and Mark Laska, Vermillion, 2001

Pilates' Return to Life through Contrology, Joseph H. Pilates, William J.Miller, Judd Robbins (ed.), Bodymind Publishing, 1998

The Pilates Workout Journal: An Exercise Diary and Conditioning Guide, Mari Winsor with Mark Laska, Perseus, 2001

Ultimate Pilates, Dreas Reyneke, Vermillion, 2002

Va Va Voom! Pilates, Yvonne Worth, MQ Publishing, 2004

Exercise videos/DVDs

Introduction to Pilates – The Power Within, IMC Vision Ltd, 2001

Isotoner Workout Volume 1, Michael King, Pilates Institute

Pilates Express, Lynne Robinson & Pat Cash, Rank Videos

Pilates Intermediate Matwork – Volume 1, Pilates Institute

Pilates Powerhouse, Body Control 5 with Lynne Robinson, Telstar Video Entertainment, 2001

Pilates, Micah Bo, International Licensing and Copyright Ltd, 2001

Pilates: The Perfect Body & Pilates Express, Telstar Video Entertainment, 2001

Pilates-Inspired Matwork – Volumes 1–3, Terra Entertainment, 2002

Super Sculpt, Michael King

Tripower, Michael King

Yogalates, Momentum Pictures Home Entertainment, 2001

Equipment

UK

Physical Company Limited, 2a Desborough Industrial Park, Desborough Park Road, Buckinghamshire, HP12 3BG
Tel. 01494 769222
www.physicalcompany.co.uk

USA

Balanced Body, 8220 Ferguson Avenue, Sacramento, CA 95828-0931
Tel. (916) 388 2838, (800) 745 2837
www.pilates.com

Australia/New Zealand

Sissel-Australia, 1 Nina Ct, Aberfoyle Park SA 5159
Tel. (08) 8322 9473
www.sissel-online.com

Index

Acknowledgements

The author and publishers would like to thank the following individuals and organizations for their assistance in the preparation of this book:

Virginia Ashworth and Patricia A. Ralston, who modelled for the photography; Sevenoaks Leisure Centre and Pilates instructor Roy Marks, who kindly allowed their Pilates classes to be photographed; Peak Pilates™ for the pictures of the Pilates machines on page 19.

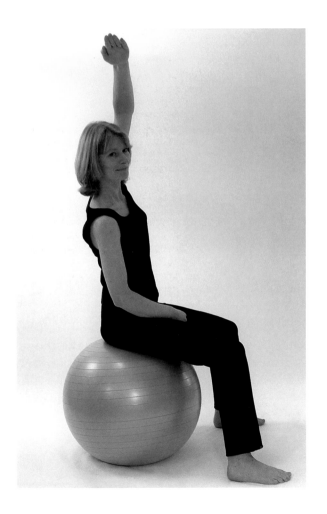

☾ Collins need to know?

Want to know about other popular subjects and activities? Look out for further titles in Collins' practical and accessible **Need to Know?** series.

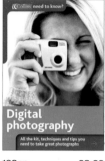

Digital photography
All the kit, techniques and tips you need to take great photographs

192pp £8.99
PB 0 00 718031 4

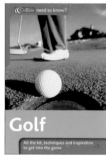

Golf
All the kit, techniques and inspiration to get into the game

192pp £8.99
PB 0 00 718037 3

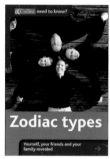

Zodiac types
Yourself, your friends and your family revealed

192pp £7.99
PB 0 00 718038 1

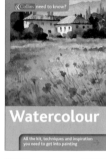

Watercolour
All the kit, techniques and inspiration you need to get into painting

192pp £8.99
PB 0 00 7189032 2

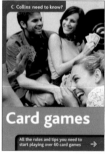

Card games
All the rules and tips you need to start playing over 60 card games

192pp £6.99
PB 0 00 719080 8

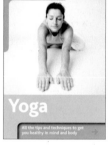

Yoga
All the tips and techniques to get you healthy in mind and body

192pp £8.99
PB 0 00 719091 3

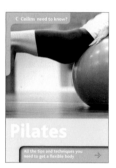

Pilates
All the tips and techniques you need to get a flexible body

192pp £8.99
PB 0 00 719063 8 8

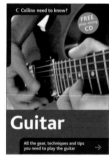

Guitar
All the gear, techniques and tips you need to play the guitar

192pp £8.99
PB 0 00 719088 3

Forthcoming titles:

Birdwatching
DIY
Drawing & Sketching
Stargazing
Weddings
French
Italian

Spanish
Kama Sutra
Dog Training
Knots & Splices
World Atlas
World Factfile

To order any of these titles, please telephone **0870 787 1732**. For further information about all Collins books, visit our website: **www.collins.co.uk**